are you
Sick
&
Tired

Dr. M. R. Swope

ARE YOU SICK & TIRED OF FEELING SICK & TIRED?

Dr. Mary Ruth Swope
P.O. Box 1746
Melbourne, Florida 32901

Copyright © 1984 by Dr. Mary Ruth Swope
Printed in the United States of America
ISBN: 0-88368-149-8

Edited by Valeria Richardson
Artwork by Loren Stiles

Special thanks to Dr. Martha Susan Brown and other faculty members of the School of Home Economics, Eastern Illinois University, for their valuable assistance.

*All Bible quotations are taken from the **King James Version** except those identified **TLB** which are taken from **The Living Bible** (Wheaton, Illinois: Tyndale House Publishers, 1971) and are used by permission.*

CONTENTS

FOREWORD

Last year, after being 50 pounds overweight for half my life, I realized I was dying. I had watched some of my friends die for some of the same reasons I was dying, and I determined that age 50 was not God's time for me to go to heaven—or wherever else fat people go when they eat themselves to death.

I also realized that simply desiring to be healthy would not get the job done. I had wanted to be healthy ever since I got fat. But each day brought the same results. Defeat.

Gradually I became aware that it takes more than desire—it takes commitment. Not just commitment to lose weight—but a commitment to change your lifestyle in regard to nutrition, exercise, and image.

The results were dramatic. And have been lasting. By proper eating and exercise I dropped from 225 pounds to 165—and there I shall stay the rest of my life.

Now, as I look back, I realized I incorporated nearly all of Mary Ruth Swope's principles into my return to life. In fact, if I were to write a book on the subject I would say all that Dr. Swope has said in these pages—only she says it not just from experience, but as an outstanding authority on nutrition.

What you're about to read can mean the

difference in life and death to you. Remember, it takes more than desire. It takes commitment. But once you've tasted life, you'll never want to go back to the way of death.

Read this—and live!

Jamie Buckingham
Melbourne, Florida

Chapter One

WHY ARE YOU SICK AND TIRED?

Does this conversation sound familiar?

"I can't believe it's Monday already. I could hardly get out of bed this morning and come to work."

"I know what you mean. The weekend was too short."

"Where's Mary?"

"She's not coming in today. She's sick again."

"Well, I'm not feeling so great myself. I hope the boss doesn't expect me to do any extra work today. I'm so tired, I can hardly drag around."

Many Americans are sick and tired, but why? We have all the modern conveniences and the most abundant food supply in the world. We are the best-informed, most widely-read nation that has ever existed. Yet, our state of health proves that something is drastically wrong.

Many factors contribute to this sick and tired feeling, but I am convinced that the way we eat is the main reason for the poor health of many Americans.

How Americans Eat

Over the past twenty to thirty years, the American way of eating has drastically changed. Many of these changes have been so gradual that we don't realize the extent or the danger of them. Our sick and tired state of health is directly related to these dietary changes. How has the American diet changed?

Whole grain, cooked cereals like oatmeal and cream of wheat are practically a thing of the past. Today, the modern breakfast consists of doughnuts, sweet rolls, boxed cereals, white toast, or pancakes. Coffee and sweetened fruit juices have replaced milk as the favorite breakfast drink.

Luncheon menus have also deteriorated. Many Americans no longer eat lunch at home. Fast-food chains, local restaurants, and school cafeterias have replaced Mom's homemade vegetable soup and fresh whole wheat bread. Hamburgers, pizza, batter-dipped chicken, and deep-fried fish have taken over as the lunchtime favorites.

The evening meal may be prepared at home, but it is very different from the dinner Grandma used to serve. We look for the most convenient way to give our families a square meal—instant potatoes, frozen meat patties, TV dinners, and canned vegetables. Our foods are refined and processed until most of the nutrients are destroyed leaving only the calories behind.

Some of the things we eat are man-made

fabrications—put together with "imitation" ingredients, additives, and preservatives. Would you call imitation mayonnaise, bacon bits, coffee creamer, whipped topping, and imitation ice cream *foods?*

What effect do these fabricated foods have on our bodies? Margarine is a man-made food that has been around for many years. It is made by adding hydrogen to oil to make it hard at room temperature. It is now a well-established fact that about 50% of the oil changes from the natural to an unnatural fatty acid form. This "trans" form has no natural metabolic function, and our bodies don't know how to handle it. The result is that it interferes with normal fatty acid metabolism.

What about the beverages we drink? Are we drinking more, or less, water and milk? Think about it. What beverages do you drink most often?

"In the past ten years, the total quantity of fluids hasn't changed much, but the type of beverage has. We have cut down on *water* (from 67 to 56 gallons per person per year), *coffee* (from 37 to 31.5 gallons), and *milk* (from 26 to 24.5 gallons). We are drinking more *soft drinks* (from 22.3 to 31.5 gallons), *beer* (from 16.5 to 21.5 gallons), *tea* (from 6.5 to 21.6 gallons), *juices* (4 to 6 gallons), *liquor* (from 1.6 to 2 gallons), and *wine* (from 1 gallon to 1.75 gallons)."[1]

The American Love Affair

Americans love sweets. We sell candy bars for

the high school band, purchase cookies from the scouts, and make chocolate-covered brownies for the class bake sale. But who cares if our children's teeth and bones are brittle and decayed? So what if blood vessels are victimized, fatty hearts are developed, and resistance to infection is lowered? It was for a good cause, wasn't it?

One of my former associates was a dental surgeon who had a three-year-old girl. Her father knew that sugar ruins teeth, so he had never permitted her to eat any candy.

At a Christmas party in their home, one of the guests brought a box of chocolates. The little girl passed the box around to the guests, then asked if she could have a piece. The father shook his head "no." A guest seated nearby said, "Oh, come on. One piece isn't going to hurt anyone. Let her have it." The father consented. I will never forget what happened.

The child put the candy in her mouth, chewed it a few times, got a puckered-up look on her face, spit it out on the floor, and said, "Ugh! What's that *horrible* stuff?"

Most children have to learn to eat highly sweetened foods. They find them unpleasant in their mouths until they develop a taste for them. Yet, from the time they are little ones, our children are given candy and sweets as prizes and rewards.

It is no wonder that "sugarholism" is now rampant in our country. In the past 100 years, sugar consumption has skyrocketed! Each person in

America eats an average of 130 pounds of sugar each year.

130 LBS. OF SUGAR PER YEAR

Diet And Disease

Have these changes in the American diet affected the state of our health? No doubt about it.

The first medical report of a heart attack appeared in a major American medical journal in 1912. Doctors didn't know what to call this new problem so they made up the term "heart attack." We are now losing *one million* Americans each year to this tragic disease.

Diabetes is an old disease. The Greeks described

it in their writings. At the turn of this century in America, however, few people had it. Today there are an estimated *8.5 million* cases with 600,000 new cases being diagnosed annually.

What about hyperactivity in children? Twenty years ago there was not one case recorded in medical literature. Doctors now estimate there are *one million* hyperactives in our nation.

Dental caries, colon cancer, diverticulitis, hypertension, osteoporosis, prostate gland problems, ulcerative colitis, breast cancer, arthritis—these are a few of the major conditions that are now epidemic in America. But they are almost unknown in underdeveloped countries where "civilized groceries" have not invaded their stores or landed on their dining tables.

Prior to 1950 a colony of Eskimos north of Canada ate a diet consisting mostly of seal, carribou, and homegrown vegetables. Then the U.S. Government built radar stations in the Eskimo territory and trained the local inhabitants to operate them. Because the men could no longer hunt and fish for their food supply, a modern grocery store was built in their community. The Eskimos began to eat the packaged and processed foods included in the typical American diet. The sugar intake of the Eskimos up to that time had been about 2 lbs. per person per year. Within five years, the Eskimos increased their sugar intake and adopted the disastrous American way of eating. Here is what happened in less than ten years:[2]

- Diabetes increased 400 percent.
- Prior to 1955 there had been no *gallbladder* surgery in the local hospital. By 1965 their gallbladder surgeries were up to U.S. figures.
- *Heart attacks* increased by 300% in ten years.
- From 1958-61, 80% of the teenagers had *acne*. No cases were reported before 1955.
- *Dental caries* became epidemic. Prior to 1950 the Eskimos did not have a local dentist because they had not needed one.
- Recurring *infections* and *anemia* in infants increased greatly.
- *Hypertension* was greatly increased.

Within ten short years of a modernized diet, there was a dramatic increase in the incidence of the degenerative diseases prevalent in developed countries like America.

Yes, the foods and beverages we eat and drink greatly affect our health.

The wife of one of my former employers began to have severe pains in her back. They grew worse and worse until she went to a physician for help. He told her (she was about 60 at the time) that she was beginning to get arthritis and with treatment she could expect to improve.

Although she followed his advice, she became so ill that she was bedridden and immobile. Finally, the family decided to take her in an ambulance to her son's home in another state. Her son, a medical doctor, examined her and found that her back was broken in two places. The bones of her

CHOICES ARE HARD!

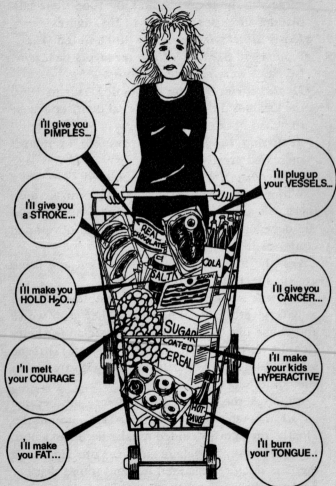

spine had literally deteriorated—crumbled. She was diagnosed as having osteoporosis (porous bones).

I will never forget what her husband told me. "You're a nutrition teacher," he said. "Tell your students about my wife's case. We have been married for nearly forty years, and I have never seen her drink a drop of milk. She ate a little bit of ice cream, now and then. For years I have been telling her that she would have brittle bones when she got older, but she wouldn't listen. Now she'll be in a cast for several months, and without a miracle she may never be able to put the weight of her body on her feet again—without crutches or a walker."

This man probably wonders why he has to suffer the consequences of his wife's habits. She will never again be able to live a normal, happy life doing all the things she had contributed to their home and marriage.

Over the past fifty years, the American diet has changed dramatically. Some changes have been good, but the overall effect has created serious health problems. The over-consumption of meat, fats, sugar, cholesterol, salt, and alcohol has been linked with a higher incidence of six of the ten leading *causes of death* in the United States: heart disease, cancer, diabetes, cerebrovascular disease, arteriosclerosis, and hypertension.

Dietary Quacks

Americans have a pill for everything. Every year we swallow millions of capsules bought at local drug stores and supermarkets. Some people think their nutrition problems can be solved by taking huge doses of certain vitamins and minerals. Others think the answer is in eating special sugar substitutes, fiber concoctions, or products bought at the health food store.

Our nutrition knowledge is limited to what we learn from TV commercials, magazines, and so-called "experts." The salespeople for most nutrition related products usually have no training in the science of nutrition. Instead, they rely on the advertisements written by their company to promote the sale of their wonder product. Many people have ruined their health or lost their lives because they carefully followed a salesman's directions.

A personal friend of mine had heard that megadoses (large amounts) of vitamin A would solve her skin problem and keep her hair from graying. Unfortunately, my friend was misled. She recently died of liver damage. Her death was primarily attributed to overdoses of vitamin A.

Many people have damaged their health because they followed the charlatans, the fakes, and the quacks of dietary misinformation. The letters M.D. sometimes follow the names of the authors of totally *unreliable* nutrition books.

with degrees in the science of nutrition from accredited universities.

Why are you sick and tired? The answer may be in your refrigerator, your grocery cart, or on your kitchen table. Look around and see if your way of eating could be the source of your physical problems.

Chapter Two

NUTRITION AND YOUR BODY

Have you ever said, "My mind isn't as quick as it used to be. I keep forgetting where I put things"?

Or, you may have heard a mother say, "Sally has had one cold after another all winter. I don't know why she's always sick."

I often hear people say, "My nerves are always on edge. I can't seem to relax."

What determines your nervous condition, how well you remember, or how effectively your body fights infection? The answer could be in your diet.

The food you eat affects four aspects of your body's performance: mental activity, nervous stability, work output, and ability to resist infections and disease.[1]

Your Mind And Memory

The quality of your diet affects your power of concentration, the speed and the depth of your comprehension, your ability to remember, and the length of your attention span. Diet also affects your ability to do what is called sustained mental

20

application and achievement (the ability to successfully "study hard" for long periods of time without extreme fatigue).

A number of studies have shown that people who live on very low-calorie diets or on diets of poor nutritional quality do not have a high level of mental performance. Studies have been done on men confined to concentration camps during World War II and on people living in countries where a substandard diet is the norm. These studies show that mental fatigue and inferior mental performance are associated with under-nutrition. However, the mind's performance gradually returns to normal when an adequate diet is restored.

We have all known older people in their nineties about whom we say, "Their mind is clear as a bell." Unfortunately, there are also many people in their sixties or seventies who have very poor memories and substandard powers of concentration. Some of the blame for this condition can be laid at the door of the quality of their lifelong food habits.

Good nutrition does result in good mental performance.

Breakfast And Better Grades

What about your children? Can a good diet help them to make better grades in school?

From controlled studies of children living on very meager diets, teachers complained of the pupils' inability to concentrate, their slowness to learn, their poor retention of subject matter, and their general inattention to school matters. When the diets of these same children were improved, these conditions were reported less frequently. Also, fewer students were retained in the same grade, and larger percentages of children were promoted to the next higher grade.

A child's poor diet is reflected in poor mental performance while a good diet has positive effects on scholastic achievement. Carefully controlled studies show that children who go to school after they have had a good breakfast perform at higher levels of scholastic achievement and have better attitudes toward schoolwork than those same children when they have no breakfast.

As a nutritionist working with hundreds of elementary school children, I observed that "no-breakfast" children were fidgety and troublesome by mid-morning. Children who had eaten a good breakfast before school were still hard at work up until the lunch bell rang.

We can conclude on the basis of research that raising the level of nutrient intake in a child's diet may very well be one way of assuring an improvement in their grades.

This conclusion also applies to adults. Improving your own state of good nutrition may restore the initiative you need to accomplish mental tasks at higher levels of performance than is possible on an inadequate diet. If you are a "no-breakfast" person, you are probably cheating yourself in terms of job satisfaction and your overall quality of health and life. You are also cheating your employer and your family!

Your Nerves And Moods

If our TV ads are a true indication of Americans' health status, millions of people must be suffering from nervousness of one kind or another. We apparently can't sleep without chemical relaxers and can't digest our food without a few pills. We need some form of stimulant to get rid of our blah moods and give us pep. Does our food intake have anything to do with these conditions?

Research studies conclude that adverse personality changes *do* occur during periods of prolonged calorie deficiency. The term used to describe this cluster of symptoms is "semistarvation neurosis." Words like irritable, restless, nervous, depressed, poorly adjusted, moody, apathetic, disoriented, sullen, melancholy, and obstinate are only a few of the many terms used to describe the nervous system symptoms related to nutrition.

Do *you* ever experience any of these conditions? Do you feel that your moods and your behavior could often be described by the terms listed above? If so, you should keep an accurate record of all the foods and drinks you consume in a three-day period. Ask a nutritionist, a dietitian, a nurse, or a doctor, to help you assess the quality of your diet. It may be possible to reverse nervous instability if it is diet related.

You can experience dramatic improvement in your nervous symptoms when your diet contains nutrients your body needs.

Nutrition And Your Job

Researchers have devised a whole series of tests to measure our motor performance. There is the grip test, the lifting test, the endurance test, and tests requiring eye-hand coordination. Strength, speed, and endurance in all of these tests were shown to vary with the quality of diet.

One group of soldiers was put on a restricted diet and compared with another group on a very nutritious diet. The scores on the performance tests of the soldiers on the inadequate diet were lower than those of the good diet group. By the end of the experiment about one-third of the original strength of the men on a poor diet was lost. After returning to a nutritious diet, the men regained their original strength within a three-month period.

Poor food habits have been shown to be associated with fatigue, physical inefficiency, and decreased work output.

One major company during World War II installed a cafeteria in its factory to provide employees the opportunity of having three good meals a day. They found that within months absenteeism declined, and the productivity of the workers was significantly increased.

Without exception, industrial workers who ate breakfast did significantly more work in the late morning hours than their co-workers who came to the factory without eating breakfast. In addition, a mid-morning snack fed to the non-breakfast group compensated for lack of breakfast for only about half of the workers in relation to the amount of work they accomplished.

A study was done by the Seventh-Day Adventists with 6,000 subjects over a nine-year period. They found that people who regularly ate breakfast had (to the surprise of some of the researchers) a mortality rate that was about three-fourths that of breakfast skippers. In other words, *in this study the breakfast skippers did not live as long as breakfast eaters*. While other factors could be involved here, such as smoking, drinking habits, etc., this is still an interesting statistic.

Beating The Common Cold

Researchers could say, "Don't ask me why, but the laboratory, clinical, and field observations show conclusively that the presence and severity of infections go hand in hand with poor diets." These relationships are especially clear-cut in developing countries where food shortages are severe.

Perhaps the presence of adequate calories and nutrients makes it possible for the body to form antibodies necessary to overcome infections. We do not fully understand the mechanism by which resistance to infections is lowered. But it is known that too high an intake of sugar decreases the activity of white blood cells. This makes it difficult for the body to fight bacteria that can cause infection and disease.

Most of us do not practice good nutrition religiously because we do not always see a direct relationship between our diet and our health. Some people seem to be careless in their food habits and go all winter without a single cold or bout with the flu. Other people are consistently conscientious about their food intake, and yet they become ill when an infectious disease hits town. Why is this?

The answer is not clear-cut, but for some reason the defenses of those who became ill were not adequate to counterattack the offender. Maybe it was because of overwork or not enough sleep. It could be the effects of a pressured and anxiety-laden environment or a dozen other things.

Regardless, the research is clear. *People who eat good diets are, in general, less likely to become ill with infections than people who eat poor diets.*

Are You Structurally Sound?

Does good nutrition make a difference in the structure of the body itself? X-ray pictures and other methods of health assessment have taught us how to determine the quality of our bones, teeth, fat, muscles, and blood. These are the major elements of body structure that doctors use as indicators of the nutritional state of our bodies as a whole. When these health indicators are studied together, their status determines how the person feels, looks, and acts.

X-rays of our *bones* disclose their nutritional status. I was impressed by a photo in a textbook[2] of the X-rays of hand skeletons of two seven-year-old boys—one of whom was undernourished. The well-nourished hand had seven carpal bones compared to two for the undernourished one. The drawings of these photographs will give you some idea of the difference.

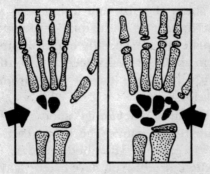

2 Carpal Centers **7** Carpal Centers

Your *teeth* are also a part of your body's bony structure. The health of your teeth is closely associated with your food intake. What foods are the worst enemies of your teeth? You would be correct if you named refined sugar in the form of

27

candy, cake icing, jelly, carbonated drinks, pies, and other sweets.

There is confirmed evidence that ordinary table sugar, as well as a combination of too many sweets of all types, causes tooth decay. Americans are eating much too much sugar. No wonder cavities are considered normal and many young adults have false teeth and dental plates.

The soft tissues of your body are also affected by your diet. The layer of fat directly under your skin protects against noise and bruising and pads the nerves. Extremely thin people are often more affected by the shrill voices of children or blaring radios than people with adequate pads of fat under their skin.

What about the size and firmness of *muscles?* Are these indicators of the quality of your health? An adequate diet, especially one that supplies all the amino acids (protein) needed for building tissue positively, affects muscle size, firmness, and coordination.

The content of our *blood* is another indicator of good nutritional status. The blood carries nutrients to all parts of your body, and it can only deliver the nutrients you have eaten. Why do doctors prick your finger or tap your veins to gain samples of blood? That is one way to obtain information about the quality and quantity of your nutrient supply. If you have a severe shortage of one or more nutrients, diagnosis of your health problem becomes easier and more certain.

Your Body Size

Body size is affected by heredity and nutrition. Inherited family characteristics have much to do with potential body build and growth. However, the dietary habits developed from infancy throughout life profoundly affect your growth and physical development.

Research shows that children in our country since the turn of this century have made substantial height gain over their forefathers. Some authors tie this fact to better economic conditions. We have had more money to spend on food, especially on the more expensive animal sources of protein. Young adults today average about two inches taller than their counterparts of sixty years ago.

This same concept has been at work in other countries, such as Japan. Present-day Japanese children are of greater height and weight than their counterparts of fifty years ago. Due to good economic times, the Japanese diet has improved in the past few decades, especially since World War II. This increase in body size has caused Japanese clothing manufacturers to change all clothing sizes to accommodate their taller, heavier population.

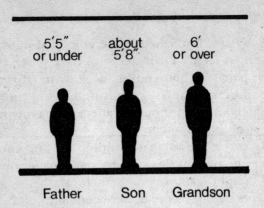

5'5" or under	about 5'8"	6' or over
Father	Son	Grandson

When I lived in San Francisco, I often observed the employees in Chinese restaurants. The grandfather who took our money at the cash register was less than 5'5" tall. His son the maitre d', who was probably born in China but partially raised in our country, was around 5'8" tall. The grandson, born and reared in the Unites States, was about 6' tall.

How Long Will You Live?

Does nutrition influence the length of your life? The U.S. Department of Health, Education and Welfare Vital Statistics show that Americans are living longer than their turn-of-the-century counterparts. Gains in longevity are undoubtedly due to a number of different factors—advances in medical science, improved public health services, better economic and social conditions. The great gains in nutrition knowledge and improved dietary habits have helped eliminate a number of conditions related to malnutrition.

Americans are living longer, but will this trend continue? *The chief causes of death in our country are thought to be diet related.* Unless we alter our food patterns to lessen the incidence of chronic degenerative diseases, there cannot be continued gains in our longevity.

One medical doctor said recently that at the beginning of this century *1 in 13* Americans had cancer; in 1982, *1 in 4* had it. He believes that by 1990 the statistic will be *1 in 3* and by the year 2000—*1 in 2*. Let's hope his predictions are inaccurate.

The *American Institute for Cancer Research Newsletter* for May 1984 said, "The top researchers in the field of diet and cancer say that a major portion—40%, 50% even 60%—of all cancer deaths in this country *could be avoided with proper changes in diet!*"

Your Dietary Lifestyle

Where do you find yourself in regard to your eating habits? Are you doing all you can to have an adequate diet? Let me encourage you to spend the time and money necessary to nourish your body well. Your own "health security" may prove to be more valuable to you than your "social security."

Because of our great affluence (and other factors in our society) we have become the "I want it now" generation. But there is no quick, easy, pain-

31

less way to good health. Pills cannot fill all of your nutritional needs. Special diets of all kinds should be considered suspect until careful study proves otherwise. Health potions cannot substitute for eating the right kinds and amounts of fruits, vegetables, cereals, meats, and milk.

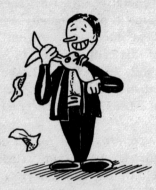

THERE IS <u>NO</u> NUTRITION **MAGIC**!

The dietary lifestyle you choose will affect your body performance, body size, resistance to disease, and your life expectancy. If you're sick and tired of feeling sick and tired, only *you* can effect the remedy. There is no magic solution!

Chapter Three

HOW TO EAT RIGHT

Do you ever think about what you are eating or why? Do you ever stop to consider if the foods you are eating contain any nutrients?

Most of us eat three meals a day without giving much serious thought to the choices we make. We eat foods that appeal to our eyes and tastebuds— not necessarily what our bodies need.

Dr. Jeffrey Bland in his book, *Your Health Under Seige,*[1] includes a questionnaire to help us assess the quality of our dietary lifestyle. The following is an adaptation of the ten items in his test, along with his suggested scores:

1. Number of times per week that you eat meals or snacks at fast-food restaurants. (For an *excellent* diet your score should be 0-1; if it is 8-10, your rating is a *poor diet*.)

2. Number of soft drinks consumed per week. (A score of 0-1 is *excellent*; 12 or more is a *very significant problem,* hereafter referred to as *V.S.P.)*

3. Meals per week with green, leafy vegetables. (Less than 5-7 is a *poor diet* score.)

4. Number of beef, pork, or lamb meals eaten per week. (0-3 is *excellent*; 4-7 is *good*; 8-10 is *moderate*; 14 or more is *V.S.P.*)

5. Number of teaspoons of sugar added to each cup of coffee, or number of candy bars consumed per week. (0-1 is *excellent*; 8 or more is *V.S.P.*)

6. Cups of coffee per day. (0-1 is *excellent*; 6-7 is *poor diet*; 8 or more is *V.S.P.*)

7. Slices of whole grain bread eaten per week. (14 or more is *excellent*; less than 5 is *V.S.P.*)

8. Number of sweet desserts consumed per week. (0-3 is *excellent*; 11-14 is *poor diet*; 15 or more is *V.S.P.*)

9. Number of meals or snacks with milk or low-fat cheese per week. (9 or more is *excellent*; 3-4 is *poor diet*.)

10. Number of days per week that you do *not* eat three *balanced* meals. (0-1 is *excellent*; 4 is *poor*; 5 or more is *V.S.P.*)

If I had designed such an evaluation test, I would have added questions such as:

1. How many meals per week do you have deep-fried foods? _____

2. How many mornings a week do you eat doughnuts, sweet rolls, pancakes, French

toast, coffee cake, or other highly sweet-ened foods for breakfast? _____

3. How many times per week are you drinking a liquid diet mix as your only food? _____

4. How many meals per day are you eating more calories than you are using through work and exercise? _____

5. How many servings of fruit do you eat daily? _____

6. How many days per week do you get 2-3 tablespoons of dietary bran? _____

For the first four items your answers should be 0-1. For items five and six, you should eat 1-2 fruits daily and 2-3 tablespoons of dietary bran every day (not crude fiber).

If you and your family are sick and tired of feeling sick and tired, then it's time to do something about it!

We all like to eat, but food is worthless if it contains no *nutrients*. Some foods are valued above others because they supply more nutrients to your body. Soft drinks are void of any nutrient except sugar. Milk, on the other hand, is so full of food value that even adults could live on milk alone—if they included foods containing iron and vitamin C.

Have you ever read the labels on packaged foods from the supermarket? The most important nutrients are listed first: *carbohydrates, protein,* and *fat. Vitamins* and *minerals* are usually listed next.

We're all familiar with vitamin C and A, but there are many others that our bodies need for good health. There are fifteen vitamins and over twenty minerals important in human nutrition. However, those numbers could change as additional nutrients are discovered.

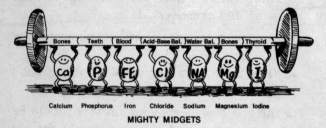

Bones	Teeth	Blood	Acid-Base Bal.	Water Bal.	Bones	Thyroid
Ca	P	FE	Cl	NA	Mg	I
Calcium	Phosphorus	Iron	Chloride	Sodium	Magnesium	Iodine

MIGHTY MIDGETS

The fact that a nutrient is needed in small amounts does not mean that its function in the body is an unimportant one. For instance, it is recommended that adults consume three micrograms of vitamin B-12 every day. (One whole gram of vitamin B-12 wouldn't even fill up a quarter-teaspoon, and we're talking about three-millionths of that!) But without that tiny amount, a very serious disease known as *pernicious anemia* can develop, causing nerve damage, paralysis, and mental retardation.

The Nutrients You Need

Nutrients do not perform their specific function alone—they work as teams. If one member is missing, the body functions will be performed poorly or the job may not get done at all. A woman I know never drank milk. When she broke her wrist in an accident, her body did not contain the proper minerals needed to heal the broken bone properly. When the bone was completely knitted, the wrist had an ugly bulge on it. Her physician explained that her body had to use second-choice nutrients because adequate amounts of calcium and phosphorus were lacking.

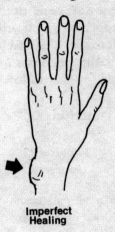

**Imperfect
Healing**

The growth and maintenance of bones depend on protein, vitamin C, vitamin A, vitamin D, calcium, phosphorus, magnesium, and flouride to mention only a few. However, it is dangerous to take individual vitamins or minerals without a doctor's supervision. Overdoses can create a shortage of other nutrients and the body can be harmed as a result.

There are six classes of nutrients: carbohydrates,

fat, protein, vitamins, minerals, and water. Their functions can be grouped into three categories:

1. Some nutrients *provide energy.*

2. Some nutrients *build, repair, and maintain* body tissue.

3. Some nutrients *regulate body processes.*

Many people are sick and tired because they do not get the proper nutrients from the food they eat. If you want to stay well and have more energy, make sure your diet includes foods listed in the nutrient information that follows.

Sources And Functions Of Selected Nutrients

Nutrient	Important Sources	Some Major Functions
Carbohydrates	cereal, potatoes, dried beans, corn, bread, sugar, pasta	Supplies energy so protein can be used for growth and maintenance of body cells.
Protein	meat, poultry, fish, milk, cheese, eggs, dried beans, peas	Supplies energy; part of every cell-muscle, blood and bone; part of enzymes, some hormones & body fluids, antibodies.

Fat	shortening, butter, salad dressings, oils, cheese, cream	Supplies energy; in every cell; provides & carries vitamins A, D, and K; provides essential fatty acids.
Vitamin A	liver, carrots, leafy greans, butter, margarine, sweet potatoes, pumpkin	Functions in visual processes; helps maintain healthy skin, thus increasing resistance to infection.
Thiamin (B_1)	whole grains, fortified cereals, nuts, dry beans	Aids carbohydrate use, promotes appetite, aids nervous system.
Riboflavin (B_2)	liver, milk, yogurt, cottage cheese, eggs, salmon, green vegetables	Aids in production of energy in cells, promotes healthy skin, vision, & eyes.
Niacin	liver, meat, poultry, fish, peanuts, cereals, whole grains	Promotes healthy skin, nerves, digestion, appetite, energy use in cells.

Vitamin C	broccoli, orange, grapefruit, papaya, mango, strawberries	Strengthens blood vessels, hastens healing, increases resistance to infection, aids in use of iron.
Calcium	milk, yogurt, cheese, collard, kale, mustard, turnip greens, sardines	Aids in building bones & teeth, in blood clotting, muscle relaxation, & nerves.
Iron	prune juice, liver, dried fruits, dried beans & peas, meats	Required for oxygen utilization, increases resistance to infection, aids in use of energy.
Phosphorus	milk products, meat, eggs, cereals, whole grains, poultry	Used with calcium in bones & teeth; regulates many body processes.
Vitamin (B_6)	liver, fish, soy and lima beans, whole grain cereals, peanuts	Helps utilize protein, fat, & carbohydrates.

Vitamin (B$_{12}$)	Only in animal foods— liver, meat, fish, shellfish, milk, milk products, eggs, poultry. Vegetarian diets should include milk or a (B$_{12}$) supplement.	Assists in the maintenance of nerve tissues and normal blood formation.
Folic Acid	Green leafy vegetables, liver, dry legumes, nuts, whole grain cereals, some fruits especially oranges	Assists in normal blood formation; helps enzymes and other biochemical systems function.
Iodine	Seafood, iodized salt	Helps regulate the rate at which the body uses energy.
Vitamin D (the sunlight vitamin)	Vitamin D milk, fish liver oils, sunshine	Helps absorb calcium from the digestive tract and build calcium and phosphorus into bone.

| Vitamin E | Vegetable oils, green leafy vegetables, whole grain cereals, wheat germ, egg yolk, butter, milkfat | Protects vitamin A and unsaturated fatty acids from destruction by oxygen. |

Calories And Energy

Most of us are familiar with the term *calories*—especially if we've ever counted them on a diet! But what are they? Calories are the amount of energy our bodies get out of the food we eat. They measure food energy.

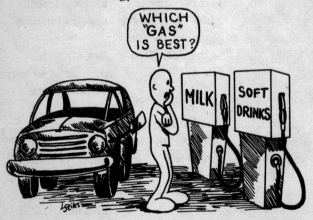

Eating food is like filling your car with gasoline. Foods provide the fuel your body needs to run on. Just as a gallon of gasoline enables your car to go a certain number of miles, food allows your body to move and function. How long it functions depends on the amount of energy (number of calories) you put into your body through the food you eat.

If you don't fill up the gas tank with fuel, the car can't start and won't run. If you don't feed your body good food, it can't function properly and won't stay healthy.

While calories are not nutrients, some nutrients do provide calories (energy). Carbohydrates, fat, and protein give your body energy because they contain calories. When you are on a diet, you count calories from foods containing one or more of those nutrients.

While vitamins and minerals do not provide calories, some B-vitamins make it possible for the body to make the best use of the energy that carbohydrates, fat, and protein provide.

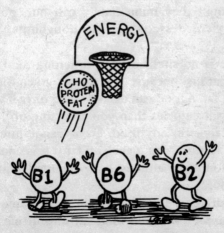

Think of it as trying to open a can of soup. You have to use a can opener to open the can to get the soup out. You don't get soup from the can opener—you get it out of the can. But you need the can opener to get to the soup. Water and some of the vitamins and minerals are like can openers. They get the energy value out of the carbohydrates, fat, and protein we eat.

Are Calories Fattening?

Most people associate calories with their weight. If a person is overweight, they have to "cut calories" to lose, or "watch their calories" in order to maintain their weight. Unfortunately, many people do not understand enough about the calorie value of food to be able to balance their energy input with energy outgo. When you ask any group of women to name the foods they think are "fattening" they immediately call out: potatoes, bread, rice, desserts, candy, doughnuts, potato chips.

There is no such thing as fattening food in the sense that just because you eat any given food you will get fat. A food can make you fat *only* if you eat more total calories than you are using up in your daily activities. Any food, even orange juice, carrots, or lettuce, can make you fat if it is consumed when you have already had your daily quota of calories.

We often fool ourselves about the amount of food we are eating. If one-half cup of ice cream has 150 calories, we forget that a cereal bowl full can have as many as 500-700! If one small dipper of blue cheese dressing has around 250 calories, then the three dippers we pour on our salad bar lunch totals around 750. One 12-ounce cola drink has about 135 calories, but four a day supplies 540 calories and a total of 36 teaspoons of sugar! The sugar adds nothing nutritional except glucose—a substance that adds stress to our system and can cause disease.

Another easy way to mount up hundreds of calories is to add butter, sour cream, and cheese to baked potatoes and other dishes. You can add as many as 350 calories to the innocent little 90-100 calorie Idaho bakie! These extras are high in fat—something known to cause hardening of the arteries and heart disease.

I have seen youngsters, and adults alike, eat a handful of chocolate chip cookies—rinsing them down with a glass of milk or a large soft drink. Want to guess how many calories you can consume that way? Don't be surprised if it is 600-750 or even more!

The average adult woman who is working in a sedentary job can eat only a total of 1500-1800 calories per day without gaining weight! Can you understand why it is so easy to gain weight on a typical American diet? Just 150 unneeded calories a day result in a weight gain of 13 pounds in a year.

A fast-food meal of a ground beef or fish sandwich with mayonnaise, French fries, and a soft drink totals from 900-1400 calories. After a lunch like that there aren't many calories left for dinner!

Variety—The Spice Of Life

You should *not* eat the same foods day after day because allergies to these foods can be developed. In addition, you can get an oversupply of some nutrients and an undersupply of others. The fact that two-thirds of the calories in the typical American diet is composed of fat and sugar explains why we are short in vitamin A, vitamin C, calcium, and iron. We need *four* one-half cup servings of fruits and vegetables every day. If we choose four servings of green beans (2 cups) to meet this recommendation, the nutrient intake would be as follows:

	Calcium	Iron	B_1	B_2	B_3	Vit. A	Vit. C
	mg	mg	mg	mg	mg	IU	mg
2 cups *green beans*	126	1.6	0.18	0.22	1.2	1360	30

If you replace two of those servings of green beans with a *potato* at each of two meals your nutrient intake improves.

	Calcium	Iron	B_1	B_2	B_3	Vit. A	Vit. C
	mg	mg	mg	mg	mg	IU	mg
1 cup *green beans*	63	0.8	0.09	0.11	0.6	680	15
2 med. *potatoes*	18	1.4	0.2	0.08	3.4	trace	40
Total	81	2.2	0.29	0.19	4.0	680	55

If you replace one serving of green beans with one-half cup of *broccoli*, you get a real bonus!

	Calcium mg	Iron mg	B_1 mg	B_2 mg	B_3 mg	Vit. A IU	Vit. C mg
½ cup *green beans*	32	0.4	0.05	0.06	0.3	340	8
2 med. *potatoes*	18	1.4	0.2	0.08	3.4	trace	40
½ cup *broccoli*	68	0.6	0.07	0.15	0.6	1940	70
Total	118	2.4	0.32	0.29	4.3	2280	118

Finally, if you substitute one potato with a *banana,*the nutrients really mount up!

	Calcium mg	Iron mg	B_1 mg	B_2 mg	B_3 mg	Vit. A IU	Vit. C mg
½ cup *green beans*	32	0.4	0.05	0.06	0.3	340	8
1 med. *potato*	9	0.7	0.1	0.04	1.7	trace	20
½ cup *broccoli*	68	0.6	0.07	0.15	0.6	1940	70
1 med. *banana*	10	0.8	0.06	0.07	0.8	230	12
Total	119	2.5	0.28	0.32	3.4	2510	110

You can easily see that variety increases the overall nutrient content of your diet. Remember all foods are not equivalent in their nutrient content—some are better sources of certain nutrients than others. *Variety is important.* Well-liked foods can be included in the diet as long as other foods are selected to make up for any nutrient deficiencies.

In addition to eating fruits and vegetables, it is important to select from the other three food groups. Milk will provide additional calcium, riboflavin, and vitamin A; meats and cereal foods will contribute additional iron and B-vitamins.

Guidelines For Eating

Do you need to change your eating habits? If so, how do you go about it?

Here is an easy chart for you to use in planning your menus and buying your groceries.

Breads and Cereals Group—4 or more servings daily.
One serving is *any* of the following:
   1 slice whole wheat or other whole grain bread
   ¾ cup cooked cereal
   1¾ cup boxed cereals (check the sugar content!)
   ¾ cup grits, macaroni, rice, spaghetti, noodles (use whole wheat products)

Vegetable-Fruit Group—4 or more ½ cup servings daily
Select one food from each of the groups listed.
Vitamin C-rich:
   oranges, cabbage, cantaloupe, broccoli, watermelon, kale, spinach, tomatoes
Vitamin A-rich:
   dark green or yellow vegetables, broccoli, carrots, kale, pumpkin, squash, chard, collards

Meat and Meat Substitute Group—2 or more servings daily
One serving is *any* of the following:

2-3 oz. of meat, poultry, or fish (not 6-10 oz.!)
1 egg (not more than 5 per week)
⅔ cup dry beans or peas (cooked)
2 tablespoons peanut butter (or other nut butters)

Milk Group—2 or more servings daily.
One serving is *any* of the following:
1 cup milk, buttermilk, or soybean milk
1 1-inch cube of cheese (cheese is high in fat)
⅔ cup cottage cheese (low fat is best)
1 cup yogurt (plain has fewer calories)

Eating three balanced meals a day is only part of the solution to your nutrition problem. Here are some additional guidelines that will contribute to improving your health and eliminating that sick and tired feeling.

1. Eat slowly and chew your food thoroughly. Most of us eat too fast, chew our food too little, and take bites that are too big for good digestion.

2. Drink enough water to keep your urine pale. The best time to drink water is before or after meals, so your digestive juices won't get diluted.

3. Do not eat between meals. Your digestion can be slowed down by several hours if additional food is eaten.

4. Eat at least 3-4 hours before bedtime. This will give time for your food to digest, and it is less likely to be turned into fat while you sleep.

5. Exercise daily. It doesn't take a lot. Exercis-

ing 20 minutes three to four days a week will help you beat that sick and tired syndrome.

6. Restrict the use of salty foods—ham, bacon, chips, salted nuts, pickles, sauerkraut. If you don't limit your salt intake, high blood pressure could be the result.

7. Eat a hearty breakfast. It will give you the energy you need to start your day and keep you going.

8. Go on a fast now and then. This will give your intestinal tract a vacation for a day or so.

9. Eat enough bran and drink plenty of water to aid in proper elimination. Colon cancer can be avoided by following this simple health rule.

10. Eat simple meals that contain only a few different kinds of food. Each food requires a specific enzyme for its digestion, and complicated meals require complicated chemistry.

What's So Great About Food?

"There must be an easier way," you may be saying. "Why can't I just take a nutrient supplement? Then I can eat what I want and still be healthy."

Taking a high-potency vitamin/mineral capsule or protein powder mix may seem like a simple solution to your nutrition problem, but is it? That's like living by the river and eating only the fish that wash up on the shore because you don't know how to fish.

Total dependence on nutrient supplements does

not teach you how to have a balanced diet or plan nutritious meals for your family. If you ever lost your vitamin pills or protein concentrate, you'd be in big trouble!

The greatest danger in dependence on manufactured products or pills is that they contribute only a few of the nutrients your body needs. Remember there are over forty nutrients presently known to be needed by our bodies. In addition, there are many unknown substances yet to be discovered and others whose value is not yet fully understood. So why take a chance on missing some vital element that you can't buy at the drug store?

Consuming nutrients in *foods* has other advantages. The process of digestion breaks down carbohydrates, fats, and proteins into small particles that the body can absorb. Carbohydrates are broken down to simple sugars, fats to simpler fat compounds, and proteins to amino acids.

Some people believe that by using special nutrient preparations they are sparing their bodies the hard work of digestion. Actually the body is more efficient at utilizing foods, which are combinations of nutrients, rather than purified preparations. The body is designed to process complex food materials, break them down *slowly,* and present them to the bloodstream from the intestines at a rate the body can best use. It has been shown that whole proteins, as contained in foods, are better utilized even by very sick, malnourished people than purified mixtures of individual amino acids.[2]

While foods contribute combinations of nutrients, many foods also contribute *fiber*. Fiber cannot be digested and used by the body, but it is important in stimulating the elimination of waste material. Without proper stimulation the intestines will become lazy and unable to function at their best. Fiber is "nature's laxative."

Our highly refined American diet lacks adequate fiber. To correct this and avoid conditions like constipation, diverticular disease, gallstones, and bowel cancer, we should reduce our consumption of low-fiber foods—meat, milk, eggs, and refined flour foods like bakery products. Eat more fiber-rich foods such as whole grains, fresh fruits, and vegetables. Two to three tablespoons of wheat bran or oat bran sprinkled on your morning bowl of cereal will meet your daily fiber needs.

Why We Need Vitamin Pills

Many changes have taken place in our American food supply and the way we eat.

—More of our foods are refined; they have less nutrients.

—We consume two to three times the recommended amount of sweets and desserts. Calories abound, but nutrients are missing.

—Snack foods and fast foods have replaced home cooking. Convenience has been substituted for nutrients.

—The time lapse from harvest to consumer is longer. This results in vitamin and mineral losses.
—Modern food preparation methods encourage nutrient loss.
—Additives to foods are detrimental to nutrient quality.

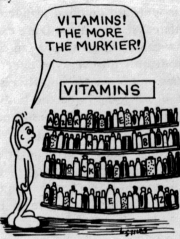

With so many factors affecting nutrient loss, most people need a nutritional supplement. If you smoke, drink, lack exercise, and live under excessive stress, you especially need a well-balanced vitamin and mineral tablet daily.

Dr. E. Reed Gaskin, M.D., an Opthamologist from Charlotte, N.C. has been impressed by the differences in his patients who have taken a vitamin and mineral supplement over a number of years and those who have not. In a letter dated

January 29, 1981, he wrote, "In my practice it seems that people who take vitamins have stronger eyes and their general physical condition is better than those who do not take vitamins."

While a vitamin/mineral supplement is good, the idea of "more is better" can be dangerous. Some nutrients are stored in the body, and if excessive amounts are ingested, dangerous levels can accumulate. Vitamins A and D are examples of nutrients that can accumulate and can cause damage or even death. However, the effects of large doses of some nutrients are not always obvious. Large doses of vitamins force the body to work overtime to get rid of what it doesn't need, causing unknown complications.

One patholigist said, "I have never examined tissue from a female brain tumor that was not flooded with vitamin B_{12}." She went on to say that in her opinion, doctors often give their patients enough B_{12} in one shot to last for five years. And yet their directions to the patient are often to come back in two weeks (or less) for another shot!

There is a range of optimal nutrient intake, below which deficiency will result but above which negative consequences can occur. What are considered safe dosages of vitamin and mineral supplements? Dr. Jeffrey Bland, Professor of Biochemistry and Nutritional Sciences of the University of Puget Sound, provides the following list to help you limit your daily vitamin and mineral intake to the proper levels.

Ranges Of Safe Daily Intakes Of
The Essential Vitamins And Minerals[3]

Vitamin A	2500-10,000 IU's
Vitamin D	200-1000 IU's
Vitamins B_1 and B_2	5-100 mg.
Niacinamide	10-1000 mg.
Vitamin B_6)	10-1000 mg.
Vitamin C	100-6000 mg.
Vitamin B_{12})	10-100 mcg.
Folic Acid	400-1000 mcg.
Pantothenic Acid	10-1000 mg.
Biotin	50-400 mg.
Vitamin E	50-1000 IU's
Iron	10-30 mg.
Copper	2 mg.
Zinc	10 mg.
Phosphorus	1000-1600 mg.
Valadium	50-100 mcg.
Manganese	2-10 mg.
Chromium	50-200 mcg.
Selenium	50-200 mcg.
Magnesium	300-600 mg.
Molybdenum	50-200 mcg.
Potassium	3000-6000 mg.
Sodium	3000-6000 mg.
Calcium	50-1200 mg.

Does stress increase your need for vitamins and minerals? There is little documented evidence that physical or psychological stress significantly increases our nutrient needs above recommended daily allowances (RDA). Illness, injury, surgery, pregnancy, and lactation *do* increase our need for certain nutrients. However, unless stress is exaggerated and prolonged, our own defense systems keep us balanced.

Here are some dietary guidelines to follow when you are under stress:

1. Eat plenty of fresh fruits and vegetables.
2. Decrease your sugar intake to as near zero as possible.
3. Avoid eating fried foods altogether.
4. Eat more bran and high-fiber foods.
5. Drink plenty of water.
6. Substitute some whole grain foods and legumes for meat.
7. Cut down on caffeine consumption.

Eating right requires planning, discipline, and determination, but the results are well worth the effort. At first you may need to refer often to the food charts and guidelines given in this chapter. But soon you will find that choosing the right foods is second nature to you—something you can't afford to live without.

Chapter Four

YOUR MONEY AND YOUR FOOD

Our supermarkets are filled with an overwhelming number of food products from which to choose. But how do we know which foods will give us the most nutrients for our money?

Protein foods (especially meats, milk, cheese, nuts) cost the most money per pound. Advertisers give us the impression that protein foods are almost magical in their qualities. We are encouraged to eat high-protein diets selected from foods and specialty products. Protein powders, bars, and drinks are promoted as necessary for a strong, healthy, beautiful body.

The first rule of efficient grocery shopping is: *Don't buy more protein than you need.* Excess protein calories are costly in dollars and cents— and to your health. This makes too much protein a double-jeopardy, pocketbook robber. Some meats have more fat than protein calories, and excess fat intake causes weight gain.

Most Americans do not lack protein in their diets. On the contrary, many consume two to three times more protein than is recommended. That is an expensive fact! Many families waste hundreds of food dollars annually on the purchase of unneeded protein foods.

Contrary to what many people think, our bodies do not require animal protein in order to be exuberantly healthy. Research supports the idea that too much protein is a major cause of premature aging and degenerative disease. Some doctors believe that excess protein causes tumorous growths and cancer. High protein intake also increases the loss of calcium from the body.

A study of vegetarian groups (Seventh-day Adventists, Chinese coolies, Hindu's, Andean Indians, and others) clearly shows their nutritional superiority. They have greater physical endurance, live longer, and have fewer diseases than those who eat meat as their chief source of protein. In addition, they lack the typical signs of early aging that meat eaters incur.

For those who are not vegetarians, research makes another important point. The body's use of protein is improved if a mixture of plant and animal proteins is consumed in the same meal. We can save food dollars and improve our nutritional status by combining meat with vegetable protein. Examples of these combinations are cereal and milk, macaroni and cheese, and the typical casserole dishes.

Many people want to cut down on meat eating,

but they do not know what to substitute for meat. Here is a very simple plan to follow:

1. Combine *grains* (wheat, rice, corn, millet, barley, rye) with *legumes* or *beans* (lentils, split peas, black-eyed peas, soybeans, pinto beans, limas, peanuts, mung beans).

2. Combine *grains* with *dairy products*.

3. Combine *legumes or beans* with *seeds and nuts* (almonds, sunflower, sesame, alfalfa, pecans, cashews, etc.). There are many delicious recipes which make use of this principle.

Comparison Shopping

Here is a chart showing the cost of different foods that provide twenty grams of protein—about one-third of what is recommended for an adult male.[1] But remember, the amount of protein is not the only factor to weigh when buying protein.

When meat prices are high, many consumers select meats like hot dogs and luncheon meats as their source of protein. But hot dogs and luncheon meats are high in fat and high in calories. The protein equivalent of four ounces of beef served in the form of hot dogs would contain almost 600 calories—an excessive amount for most of us. Select your protein foods with care—there is more to it than first meets the eye!

Comparative Cost Of Selected Sources Of Protein[2]

Food	Calories	Cost of 20 gms. of Protein
Beans, navy	300	$0.13
Peanut butter	460	.17
Bread	620	.18
Beef liver	170	.20
Eggs	250	.20
Chicken	160	.24
Hamburger	230	.25
Milk, whole	370	.25
Cheese	320	.35
Ham	130	.40
Frankfurters	490	.50
Sirloin steak	120	.60
Perch	240	.66
Bologna	500	.67
Veal cutlets	100	.70
Bacon	450	.99
Lamb chops	110	1.09

Buying Fruits And Vegetables

Fresh produce is nearly a thing of the past for most of us. Our production, distributing, and packaging processes are highly technical and extremely complicated. Yet, we are suffering nutritional and monetary losses compared to the time when most of our foods came directly from barns or backyard gardens!

You may ask, "Should I pay the higher prices for fresh produce or use canned, frozen, or dried fruits and vegetables?"

If you were to pick a fresh fruit or vegetable, undamaged, at its peak of maturity, and compare it with frozen and canned forms of the same food, the fresh product would rank highest in nutritional value. Frozen would rank second and canned third (the prolonged heat treatment in the canning process destroys some nutrients).

The cost and nutrient content of fruits and vegetables is influenced by several factors: the type of food, how old it is, the season of the year, where it was grown, and the type of processing used.

Many fruits and vegetables are picked at their peak of maturity and rushed to nearby processing plants and quickly frozen. Such frozen products would be higher in nutritional value than their fresh counterparts which travel several days to the supermarket. Fresh fruits and vegetables may be both cheaper and more nutritious at their growing site than the same products shipped long distances. Fruits and vegetables picked green and allowed to ripen on their way to distant markets do not develop their maximum nutrient content.

The effect of processing on the nutrient content and cost of a food will depend on the type of processing, the particular nutrient of concern, and the nature of the food itself. Consider the following evaluation of different foods, all of which are considered to be good sources of vitamin C.[3]

Food	Vitamin C
4 oz. Orange Juice (½ cup)	
Fresh	62mg.
Frozen, reconstituted	60
Canned, unsweetened	50
Dehydrated, reconstituted	55

4 oz. Broccoli

Fresh, raw	128mg.
Fresh, boiled	102
Frozen, boiled	82

4 oz. Potato

Raw, peeled	23mg.
Baked, or boiled in skin	17
French fried, *fresh*	28
French fried, *frozen*	18
Chips	20
Dehydrated, flakes, prepared	6
Dehydrated, granules, prepared	4

4 oz. Spinach

Fresh, raw	58mg.
Fresh, boiled	32
Frozen, boiled	22
Canned	16

There is little difference, for example, between fresh, frozen, or reconstituted orange juice. Notice that dehydrated potatoes may save you time in preparation, but processing has almost eliminated the vitamin C content. Canned spinach has half the vitamin C of cooked, fresh spinach.

Cooking For Keeps!

The way food is prepared at home will affect the nutritional value of the food you buy. In some areas, fresh greens are not considered "done" until they have cooked for at least two or three hours! The canned vegetable, on the other hand, would have been heated quickly and eaten promptly. Thus, it is possible that some fresh fruits and vegetables would actually have fewer nutrients by the time they are eaten than their processed counterparts.

It is not enough to bring the nutrients home from the store or out of the garden. The idea is to get them into the body! Here are a few guidelines for preserving the nutrients you pay for:

—Store food for only short periods of time in appropriately cool environments.

—Peel and cut foods as little as possible.

—Avoid soaking.

—Use only small to moderate amount of water in cooking.

—Consume cooking liquids.

—Avoid overcooking.

The nutrient value of vegetables depends on which part of the plant is being eaten—leaf, stem, flower, fruit, seed, tuber, bulb, or root. In general, vegetables are good sources of minerals, vitamins, and fiber but low in calories. The seed vegetables, such as corn, peas, and beans, are distinctively different from others because of their high protein content.

While vegetable protein is not considered complete by itself, it can support growth when combined with even small quantities of meat, milk, cheese, eggs, grains, nuts, or other lentils. Seed vegetables are also relatively high in calories, and their starch is well utilized by the body. With care-

ful planning a vegetarian diet can be very healthful.

Vegetables are an important food group and
should be widely used all year round—more than
just as raw salads or as a side dish.

Convenience Versus Time

What is a convenience food? A broad definition
would be any food that is partially or completely
prepared for use when it is purchased. That would
include the majority of food products in today's
supermarkets. Many food items have become so
well accepted that people no longer think of them
as convenience foods. A loaf of bread is a good
example—after all, it would have certainly been a
convenience food to great-grandmother!

Most people today, however, think of convenience foods as frozen food products like boil-in-
bag vegetables, TV dinners, frozen desserts, or
cake mixes.

Convenience means time-saving. But there can
be a nutritional and monetary cost for that saving
of time. There are several things to consider when
evaluating convenience foods and those prepared
"from scratch."

First, compare the *cost* on a per serving basis.
You can do this by adding the cost of the ingredients used in a recipe and dividing the cost by the
number of servings.

A second consideration is *time*. How much time
will actually be saved by using a convenience

food? Some may be more convenient than others! How do you value your time? There may be times when the added cost in cents is worth the time saved in preparation.

Finally, there is the *nutritional* consideration. You don't want to be short changed from a health standpoint for the price of convenience. Take for example TV dinners or frozen meat pies. While government regulations generally require a minimum amount of meat in these types of products, that amount may be much less (less than 2 ounces in some cases!) than a serving of a home prepared meal.

Certain convenience products, like specialty-type frozen vegetables, may contain added salt and sugar, which some people need to avoid. Take advantage of nutrition labeling and lists of ingredients to help you evaluate nutritional value.

The Fast-Food Phenomenon

Fast foods are now available at supermarkets, office buildings, hospitals, shopping malls, and even school lunch cafeterias. They are becoming more and more a part of the American eating pattern.

Fast foods are not the nutritional and economic bargain many people think they are. It is estimated that the cost of fast foods is about *twice as much* as similar food prepared at home.[4]

The nutritional value of a fast-food meal depends on what you select. Fast food is not necessarily junk food. However, it is typically high in calories, salt, and saturated fat. Most fast foods are also low in fiber and vitamin A. These disadvantages could affect your health if you ate at a fast-food chain everyday. Nevertheless, a typical meal of burger, fries, and shake does provide protein, B-vitamins, vitamin C, vitamin D, calcium, and iron.

Beverages often contribute a major proportion of the calories in a typical fast-food meal. Iced tea without sugar may provide two calories, compared to a large chocolate malt with as many as 840 calories!

A Big Mac, shake, and fries contain about 1,070 calories. Substituting a glass of milk for the shake and a salad for the fries greatly improves the nutrient content. Removing the high-calorie, fat-filled, batter coating on fried chicken or seafood items is another way to eliminate many unneeded calories.

Natural And Organic Foods

The recent interest in nutrition has led to an explosion of health food stores in America. These stores offer many good foods that are free of the harmful additives and preservatives often contained in supermarket brands. Health food stores also carry many whole grain flours and other unrefined food products that provide essential nutrients not found in refined and processed foods. However, any food can be classified as a *health food* if it provides nutrients the body needs.

The shopper must be wary of so-called "organic" and "natural" foods. *Organic* generally refers to the way a food is grown—without pesticides or chemical fertilizers. *Natural* is used to imply something about the characteristics of the food ingredients—that a food has no additives or artificial preservatives. Many people think if they buy organic or natural foods from a health food store, those products are superior to supermarket foods.

The scientist would define an *organic* food simply as one that contains the chemical element *carbon*. Vitamin C, for example, has a certain, specific chemical structure which contains carbon. Therefore, vitamin C is an organic compound. If it is vitamin C, it always has the same structure, regardless of where it comes from. Your body doesn't recognize the source of the vitamin C you put into it. Vitamin C is vitamin C, whether it comes from an orange or a tablet synthesized in a chemist's laboratory. Remember, however, there is an advantage to getting your vitamin C from *foods*. The food provides a mixture of nutrients, whereas the vitamin C tablet provides only vitamin C.

"Organically grown" plant foods are promoted as being nutritionally superior to those grown with chemical fertilizers. In fact, all fertilizers, whether they come from the barnyard or the farm supply store, are composed of chemicals. The plant doesn't recognize the source of the fertilizer—it simply responds in growth to the presence or absence of the chemical compounds it needs for growth. There may be good and poor organic fertilizers as well as good and poor chemical fertilizers. To claim that a plant grown organically is nutritionally superior to one grown with chemical fertilizers is misleading.

Advertising Gimmicks

Natural foods are not necessarily better for you, nor are they even necessarily natural! Many nutrient preparations are advertised as being better for you because they are "natural."

Tablets containing "rose hips vitamin C" somehow convey to the customer that a "natural" vitamin C source is better than the standard pharmaceutical tablet. In this case, if the rose hip tablet contained only rose hip vitamin C, it would be as big as a golf ball, because rose hips have such a small percentage of vitamin C. In fact, synthetic vitamin C is added to the rose hip tablet and actually makes up more of the preparation than the plant-derived vitamin.[5] Many nutrient preparations are not as "natural" as the label would have you believe.

Don't be misled by advertising. A recent *Consumer Reports* magazine article[6] on "natural" and "organic" foods reported a comparison of two brands of tomato sauce. The two brands, in identical size cans, were located side by side on the store shelf. The "natural" brand claimed to have no citric acid, sugars, preservatives, artificial colors, or flavors. The store's house brand of sauce likewise did not contain those substances, but that was deemed hardly worth noting on the label because tomato sauce almost *never* contains such substances. The two brands were essentially identical except for *price*. The "natural" brand, at 85, cost almost three times as much as the store brand at 29.

What about the "natural" granola-type cereals? Consider the comparison of a conventional cereal to "*Quaker 100% Natural*" granola.[7]

	Quaker 100% Natural	Cheerios
Serving Size	1 oz. (¼ cup)	(1 oz. 1¼ cups)
Calories	120	110

Percentage Of U.S. Recommended Daily Allowances		
Protein	— 2	6
Vitamin A	*	25
Vitamin C	*	25
Thiamin (B_1)	2	25
Riboflavin (B_2)	*	25
Niacin	2	25
Calcium	2	4
Iron	2	25
Vitamin D	*	10
Vitamin B_6	**	25
Vitamin B_{12}	*	25

*contains less than 2% of USRDA for this nutrient
**value not given, but may be presumed low

Notice the serving size of the two cereals. If you eat a cup of cereal, you will get almost 500 calories in the granola but fewer nutrients in comparison to Cheerios. The amount of fruits and nuts in a serving of granola is of minimal significance to the diet. The sweeteners (usually honey or brown sugar) are often the second largest ingredient, yet offer no significant health advantage over ordinary white sugar.

Use nutrition labeling and the list of ingredients on food labels to help you evaluate the foods you buy. Don't be taken in by pretty packages or misleading terms when spending your food dollars for nutritional value.

Getting Your Money's Worth

Many people are tempted to buy food in quantity at today's prices so they won't have to buy at tomorrow's higher prices. Whether that is good "nutrinomics" depends on the food item and the method of storing.

Long-term storage requires special handling or processing, such as refrigeration, freezing, canning, drying, or freeze-drying. Such special processing has accompanying costs which must be carefully considered *before* purchase.

Consider the cost of different forms of milk. A recent trip to the grocery store provided the following prices:

	Price per cup
Fresh *whole milk* purchased as:	
Quart	16.3ᶜ
Half gallon	13.9
Gallon	12.9
Evaporated milk	16.9
Fresh *skim milk* purchased as:	

Quart	15.8
Half gallon	12.9
Gallon	10.6
Nonfat dry milk	8.7

Buying fresh milk by the gallon is obviously more economical. But if half of it spoils before you can drink it, it is no bargain at all! Evaporated milk, though more expensive per serving than fresh fluid milk, can be stored without refrigeration before the can is opened. Non-fat dry milk is less expensive than fresh skim milk and also has the advantage of not requiring refrigeration. However, there may be flavor deterioration if powdered milk is stored in a hot pantry or if it stored for too long a period of time.

Special processing, such as freeze-drying, may be expensive, but the food's nutritional value is preserved. Freeze-dried foods appear to retain their quality for years, and the simple addition of water is all that is required for their preparation.

You can take advantage of food specials and buy in quantity. However, it is not economical to buy more than can be used within a reasonable period of time. Deteriorated foods represent a loss of both money and nutrients.

Few *frozen* products are at peak quality after a year. *Dried* or low-moisture products (such as grains) can be stored for years *if* precautions are taken to prevent insect infestation or exposure to moisture and air. Most *canned* products have an extensive shelf life *if* the container remains undamaged and they are stored in a cool environment.

Getting your money's worth takes planning and practice. Take advantage of the nutrition information available to you. Remember that advertising is designed to sell products, and misleading terms and information are often used to attract buyers. Determine your nutrient needs and plan your shopping to meet those needs at the lowest cost.

Chapter Five

LET'S GO TO THE SOURCE

Can you imagine Jesus having diabetes, hypertension, or coronary heart disease? Of course not! Jesus lived in a constant state of divine health—partly because of His disciplined habits of proper eating and drinking. He also lived at a time when the limited supply of food kept Him from overeating, and strict dietary laws kept Him from being ill.

The ancient people of Israel used the Old Testament dietary laws as their nutrition sourcebook. Based on it and it alone, the Jews held firm beliefs about what was right to eat and what was wrong.

Because we have an abundance of available food today and no dietary laws to follow, each person must decide for himself how he is going to eat. If you're sick and tired of feeling sick and tired, maybe you should consider following some of the rules Jesus practiced.

The Seed-Bearing Plants

According to Jewish law all *fruits* and *vegeta-*

bles were permitted to be eaten. This was based on Genesis 1:29, "And look! I have given you the seed-bearing plants throughout the earth, and all the fruit trees for your food" (*TLB*).

About twenty *fruits* are mentioned by name in the Bible. Apples, apricots, grapes, figs, and pomegranates are mentioned more often than the caper, carob, citron, date, mulberry, olive, palm, and lemon.

Fig trees or figs are mentioned fifty times in the Bible. A healthy fig tree bore fruit about ten months out of the year in Palestine. Undoubtedly, Jesus would have had wide access to this fruit. In one of His most familiar parables, He used the fig tree to help make His point.

Dried fruits are mentioned in several different Bible passages. Raisins, figs, and dates were dried and pressed into small cakes. They were apparently made especially to be eaten while people were traveling or working away from home.[1] These dried fruits were high sources of energy and good sources of certain minerals. In addition, they were sanitary, easy to eat, and had good keeping quality.

Jesus probably ate dried fruit as He walked along the back roads and pathways of Galilee as a boy. On His first long journey to Jerusalem at the age of twelve, His mother may have taken along a good supply of dried fruit cakes.

No Limitations

What do we mean by the word *vegetable?* A college textbook defines the term as any herbacious plant whose fruit, seeds, roots, tubers, bulbs, stems, leaves, or flower parts are used for food.[2] This means that fruits, cereals, nuts, and herbs are actually vegetables, yet we do not classify them as such today. For our purposes, we will think in terms of the traditional classification of vegetable plants—green beans, onions, beets, potatoes, etc.

According to the Jewish dietary laws, all vegetables were permitted as food. But only the following vegetables are mentioned in the Bible by name: beans, corn, cucumbers, garlic, gourds, lentils, onions, and leeks.

There were no limitations on the method of cooking or serving vegetables. They could be eaten with either meat or milk products. Today's frozen broccoli with cheese sauce or escalloped potatoes would have qualified as kosher in the home of Jesus.

The Bible mentions corn more than any other vegetable. However, the word *corn* was used in the Bible to include cereal-type grains of various sorts. It is known that fresh corn, full ears in the husks, was served in Bible times. Jesus' noon meal at the carpentry shop may have included boiled corn on the cob or parched corn from a leather pouch. Parched grains of all kinds were commonly eaten in Israel.

We know that Jewish families ate vegetable and meat stews called *pottage* in the Bible. (See 2 Kings 4:38,39.) Dried legumes and grains were often cooked together with the added flavor of spices and dried fruits. Beans and lentils were also cooked with onions and spices in a variety of dishes. On feast days these foods were served with milk or cream products.

God wisely provided all the seed-bearing plants and fruits for food. His reason for doing so becomes apparent when we study the nutrient values of peas, beans, nuts, seeds, fruits, vegetables, and cereals. They contain all nutrients, in addition to the calories we need for energy. These foods are often good sources of fiber needed for the important process of elimination. Good elimination reduces the possibility of our suffering some of the common intestinal diseases, including diverticulosis and bowel cancer.

What Does Kosher Mean?

Jewish laws were very strict about which kinds of meat could be eaten and the way they were to be prepared. In Genesis 7:2, the Lord said to Noah: "Of every *clean* beast thou shalt take to thee by sevens, the male and his female; and of beasts that are *not clean* by twos, the male and his female."

The terms used to describe meats were "clean"

(tabor) and "unclean" (tame). Today the common word for permitted foods is *kosher*—a Hebrew word which means suitable, correct, or proper.

Deuteronomy 14:3-7 helps our understanding by defining *clean animals*. They are the plant-eating animals (wild or domestic) that chew the cud. "These are the animals you may eat: the ox, the sheep, the goat, the deer, the gazelle, the roe-buck, the wild goat, the ibex, the antelope, and the mountain sheep. Any animal that has cloven hooves and chews the cud may be eaten, but if the animal doesn't have both, it may not be eaten. So you may not eat the camel, the hare, or the coney" (*TLB*).

Swine are also mentioned as an animal that should not be eaten. Although it has cloven hooves, it does not chew the cud. "You may not eat their meat or even touch their dead bodies; they are forbidden foods for you" (Leviticus 11:8 *TLB*).

Jesus would not have eaten pork in any form—not even barbecued or grilled on an open pit! (See Deuteronomy 14:8.) Our favorites of baked ham, broiled pork chops, fresh pork with sauerkraut, or even the famous BLT (bacon/lettuce/tomato) sandwich would all have been "unclean" to Jesus.

Why did God forbid the eating of meat from swine? It could be because pork is high in fat and difficult to digest. It is also a source of disease when it is not cooked properly. Pigs and hogs are carriers of *trichina*—a parasitic worm found in their intestinal tract. Seven out of ten persons who use pork products are reported to have antibodies to trichina organisms in their bloodstream. This means that at some time in their lives they have had a trichina infection.[3] It seems the biblical admonition against pork is a valid one.

Meat And Milk Don't Mix

Not only were there lists of kosher and non-kosher animals, but there were also approved and unapproved methods of preparing them. (See Exodus 23:19 and Deuteronomy 14:21.) The Jews were told plainly not to cook or to eat a young goat boiled in its mother's milk. "Milk," according to Jewish definition, includes all dairy products, such as cheese, sour cream, butter, and fresh cream.[4]

In addition, a time interval of as little as one hour and as much as six hours must elapse between the eating of meat and dairy dishes.[5] While the reason for these laws is not clear, such a practice would limit the amount of saturated fat consumed in any given meal. In any event, it is almost certain that Jesus never tasted such popular American dishes as beef stroganoff, chicken a la king, creamed tuna, or dozens of other favorite recipes in which we mix meat with cream sauce containing milk, sour cream, or cheese.

Rare, Medium, Or Well-Done?

Another Jewish law had to do with the blood contained in meat. Blood is a known carrier of bacteria and spores of infectious disease. Those who eat raw blood (rare steak, for example) increase their possibility of getting sick.

Deuteronomy 12:23-25 says it this way, "The restriction is never to eat the blood, for the blood is the life, and you shall not eat the life with the meat. Instead, pour the blood out upon the earth. If you do, all will be well with you and your children" (*TLB*).

Every aspect of this law was carefully observed. The Jewish slaughtermen were a very select group of pious men who knew the Jewish ceremonial laws, as well as all of the rules regarding foods to be served at feasts and festivals. They had to pass an examination in order to obtain and keep their jobs.[6] It was their responsibility to make the flesh of the animals as bloodless as possible and not let one bit of blood congeal within the muscle. This practice had many hygienic benefits.

What about today? Would we be better off not to eat meat that contains uncooked blood? I will answer the question this way: *The only two Jewish dietary laws which were not revoked by the coming of Christ are the eating of strangled meats and the eating of blood.* (See Acts 15:19,20.)

Adam Clarke in his Bible commentary presents a very complete dissertation concerning the unlawfulness of eating blood. He concludes, "And thus we see that man had no right to the blood of the creatures before the flood; he had no right after this. . .and no man had a right to it from any concession in the law of Moses."[7] Has any such permission been given under the gospel? He concludes that there has not, but rather the direct contrary, as is shown in Acts 15.

Then And Now

How would a cook in Jesus' day have prepared meat? It could be either broiled, boiled, or fried. Meat was *broiled* over or under a flame with some kind of grill arrangement so that the fat drippings did not remain in contact with the meat. In *boiling,* the meat was cooked until the flesh fell off the bones—thus, assuring that there was no "pink flesh" to be served at the table.[8]

The Jews never fried meat in a pan containing fat and never without any way of draining off the blood as it cooked. Our method of coating the outside pieces of meat with a batter and then either pan-frying or deep-frying them in oil, lard, or hydrogenated fat is definitely not kosher. Fat absorption of the batter presents a potential health problem, especially for those who frequently eat foods prepared this way.

Deep-fried foods lie in the stomach for long periods of time causing undue stress in the process of digestion and absorption. (It can cause hours of burping!) These foods are one of the culprits thought to cause clogged blood vessels which can lead to strokes and sudden death.

The priests of Bible times were known to have eaten too much meat. This is easily understood when one studies the animal sacrificial offerings required by religious law in those times. The priests received their share of the flesh of the animals in five main offerings. Unfortunately, they earned a bad reputation for living a self-indulgent life and often suffered from obesity and gout.[9]

Many Americans are also suffering physically because of our over-consumption of meat. According to research studies, a high-protein diet can put stress on the liver, break down protein tissues, trigger a loss of calcium from the bones, and leave toxic residues which must be eliminated.[10] [11] For optimal health, therefore, high-protein diets largely from animal sources are not recommended.

The ordinary Jewish family ate meat at the most once a week.[12] Dr. Osee Hughes of Ohio State University concluded from years of study that *three servings* (4 oz. each) of meat per week were adequate to meet the protein needs of the average adult if beans, lentils, cereals, milk, cheese, eggs, and nuts were eaten in other meals.

Kosher Eggs

Both Leviticus 11:13-19 and Deuteronomy 14:12-18 list twenty "unclean" birds. Included are all birds of prey, like the vulture, hawk, and raven. The ostrich, seagull, owl, pelican, stork, eagle, and bat are also among those excluded as edible.

The Bible does not give a list of "clean" birds, so Jewish law on this point varies from community to community. Some rabbis permit the eating of turkey and pheasant while others do not.

The Bible doesn't say anything about eating *eggs,* but Jewish law is specific on this point. No eggs from "unclean" birds may be eaten because they come from an unclean source. The eggs of "clean" birds may be eaten as long as they do not contain blood spots or have not been fertilized.

Eggs were used in several feast day menus and were given to mourners on the first day of the loss of their loved one. (Could this be the source of the traditional Easter egg?) They were considered by Jews to be a very nutritious product and were served with milk, honey, and wine in many different recipe combinations.

Fins And Scales

What about *fish?* Does the Bible label them as "clean" or "unclean?" Leviticus 11:9-12 says, "As to fish, you may eat whatever has fins and scales, whether taken from rivers or from the sea; but all other water creatures are strictly forbidden to you. You mustn't eat their meat or even touch their dead bodies. I'll repeat it again—any water creature that does not have fins or scales is forbidden to you" (*TLB*).

If we were to follow the Jewish laws observed in the home and community in which Jesus grew up, we would have to change our eating patterns. We would need to eliminate from our diets all oysters, lobster, crabs, shrimp, clams, catfish, sturgeon, swordfish, and eel.

According to the Bible, the kosher fish are those which have fins and scales in the waters, in the seas, and in the rivers. (See Leviticus 11:9 and Deuteronomy 14:9.) Only fish with bony skeletons, of which there are some 30,000 varieties, are included in this definition.

The nutritive value of poultry and fish is similar to that of beef, but the fat and cholesterol content of these two foods is lower. If you remove the skin from chicken, you can eliminate much of the fat. Poultry and fish are also considerably lower in calories than beef and usually cheaper in price.

The Staff Of Life

The diet of Jesus would certainly have included the staff of life—*bread*. In fact, bread was the single most important item in His diet. To eat bread literally meant, in Hebrew and Greek, "to take a meal."[13] For most Americans eating bread is merely a supplement—we can take it or leave it.

The popular bread in the time of Jesus was far superior in nutritional quality over that of bread today. *Jewish bread* was a *whole grain* with none of the parts of the grain removed or altered by the use of modern chemicals or manufacturing

ENDOSPERM

CONTAINS ABOUT:

70-75% of the protein
43% of the pantothenic acid
32% of the riboflavin
12% of the niacin
6% of the pyridoxine
3% of the thiamine

B-COMPLEX VITAMINS

BRAN

CONTAINS ABOUT:

86% of the niacin
73% of the pyridoxine
50% of the pantothenic acid
42% of the riboflavin
33% of the thiamine
19% of the protein

GERM

CONTAINS ABOUT:

64% of the thiamine
26% of the riboflavin
21% of the pyridoxine
8% of the protein
7% of the pantothenic acid
2% of the niacin

Kernel of Wheat

processes. Because of this, the bread was dark in color, heavy in texture, very nutritious, and full-flavored. It probably contained no cane sugar, though perhaps a little honey, and no preservatives. It was made daily from freshly ground flour, with oil, and just a bit of salt added to improve the flavor.[14]

It is easy to see from the drawing[15] that when the bran and germ are removed in the milling process it results in a drastic reduction of the mineral, vitamin, and roughage content of the whole grain. If we ate whole-grain bread instead of white refined loaves, we would add much needed fiber to our diets to aid in elimination and help prevent certain diseases of the intestines which are common today.

The prophet Ezekiel had an interesting bread recipe. He said God told him to use the following ingredients: wheat, barley, beans, lentils, millet, and spelt. (See Ezekiel 4:9.) A bread product resulting from a mixture of these ingredients is high in protein, carbohydrates, vitamins (especially B_1 and B_2) and minerals (especially iron). A modern version of this recipe is available.[16]

The protein present in cereals, beans, and lentils is of the incomplete type. This means that it will not support maximum growth when consumed by humans or animals, without the aid of other protein foods. Nonetheless, when certain incomplete protein foods are used in combination with each other (as in Ezekiel's beans and grains bread) or with other protein foods like milk, cheese, meat, or eggs, they satisfy our need for complete proteins.

Milk, Cheese, And Butter

The Promised Land was flowing with milk and honey. (See Exodus 3:8.) According to Bible scholars, that statement can be taken literally. The majority of the milk produced and used in Israel was that of sheep, camels, and goats. *Camel's milk* mixed with three parts of water was one of the most popular beverages in those times.[17]

Cheeses were made from the milk of several animals. Soured milk which formed hard lumps was dried in the sun, and curds produced were used in cooking. (See Job 10:10.) Softer cheeses were made in Bible times in cloth bags in which the whey separated out and left the soft curds on the inside of the bag.[18] This was similar to what we call cottage cheese. The word *butter* is used to describe different products in the Bible. In certain contexts it means curdled milk or cream. It also could have meant the product obtained by the churning of milk—the product we think of when we hear the word butter.[19]

In a Jewish home, meat dishes could not be prepared, cooked, or served with butter because it is a dairy food. But it was kosher to serve butter with bread and on all vegetables not served with meat.

Some Oil But No Fat

The shortening most often referred to in the Bible is *olive oil,* but the eating of animal fat was to be avoided. An example of this rule is found in Leviticus 7:23 which says, "Speak unto the children of Israel, saying, Ye shall eat no manner of fat, of ox, or of sheep, or of goat." These were, you remember, the kosher meats.

Leviticus 7:25 has a further word about this matter: "Anyone who eats fat from an offering sacrificed by fire to the Lord shall be outlawed from his people" (*TLB*).

The overall fat content of the American diet now averages about 40% of our total calories—a figure well above the suggested desirable intake of around 25-35%. Total fat intake, animal fat intake, and cholesterol intake increases your risk of heart disease. A decrease in the calories you eat from fat sources (especially from animal sources) would lessen the risk of heart attack, arteriosclerosis, and strokes.

If we were to decrease our consumption of saturated fats, we would need to eat less fat meat. Lamb, pork, and beef, in that order, are the highest in fat content of our most commonly used meats.

In addition, we need to curtail our intake of butter, cream, egg yolks, cheese, whole milk, hydrogenated margarines, shortenings, coconut oil, and goods made from such products. We should also eat less fried foods, especially deep-fat fried ones, such as french fries, potato chips, fish, pies, doughnuts, etc.

Sugar Or Honey?

The only sweetener used extensively in the time of Christ was honey. Cane sugar (regular white, table sugar) was not used for food until around the fifteenth century.[20] In fact, cane sugar is not even mentioned in the Bible.

Are there any benefits to eating honey rather than sugar? Authorities are not in agreement on the nutritional benefits of honey. Dr. Jean Mayer, one of the nation's foremost authorities on nutrition, said, "Despite claims of superior nutritional benefits by honey lovers, the fact is that honey, like other sugars, is virtually devoid of other nutrients."[21]

On the other hand, an article in the *Journal of Nutrition* says that honey contains minute amounts of many vitamins and minerals. This research also shows that the nutrients in honey vary according to the color (darker ones are most nutritious) and the locality from which it comes.[22]

While the nutrients present in honey are in trace amounts, this nutritional benefit does not accrue when we consume cane sugar—a product devoid of any vitamin, mineral, or amino acid. The addition of sugar (whether white or brown) or liquid sweeteners (such as honey, molasses, corn syrup) is entirely unnecessary in meeting our nutritional needs. Nature has provided us with many delicious foods which have an excellent combination of starch, sugar, fiber, vitamins, minerals, and protein. Refined white sugar contains no nutrients—just empty calories.

Something To Drink

Water was scarce in many parts of the Middle East and often considered impure, especially in the towns and villages. To compensate for this, the Israelites drank the juice from grapes, apples, dates, corn, honey, pomegranates, and other fruit. They especially drank grape juice, which is high in calcium and contains other nutrients.

How does grape juice compare in nutritive value to today's soft drinks? Grape juice is much more healthful than any of the colas or other soft drinks consumed by Americans. *Soft drinks are empty calories* that contribute only simple carbohydrates (sugar) to our diets without the addition of a single nutrient. Our health is bound to be adversely affected if we drink large quantities of soft drinks.

The beverages that Jesus drank contributed more to His health and nutrition than the modern-day beverages we drink. Jesus was fortunate to have lived in a time when the main beverage choices were milk, water, or fruit juices. Fortunately, we can still make the same choices today—*if* we want to be healthy!

Eating The Bible Way

The Jews generally ate two daily meals: breakfast and supper. (See Luke 14:12; John 21:12.) The first meal was usually light, consisting of milk, cheese, bread, or fruits, and eaten at various hours from early morning to the middle of the forenoon. In the early history of the Israelites, the principal meal, corresponding with our dinner, was eaten about noon. (See Genesis 43:25.) At a later period, at least on festive occasions, it was taken after the heat of the day was over. This was supper.[23]

It is not God's fault that many of us are sick, undernourished, and unhealthy. God originally supplied every part of the world with a proper balance of foods and nutrients to sustain the local inhabitants. Man-made customs and cultural traditions are responsible for the mistakes which have led to nutrition-related disease and suffering.

The science of nutrition will never prove that God was ignorant about or negligent in supplying the perfect types, amounts, or proper combinations of nutrients to meet man's requirements for abundant health. However, many of *us* are ignorant of our nutritional requirements and negligent in supplying our bodies with these nutrients.

Do you think God is interested in your diet or were His rules designed only for earlier generations? God loves you and wants you to live a long and healthy life. If you follow the guidelines He has established in His sourcebook, the Bible, you will live an abundant life according to His perfect plan.

Chapter Six

HOW YOUR DIET AFFECTS
YOUR HEALTH

Cancer, diabetes, heart attack—these words strike fear into the minds of many Americans. We all know friends and relatives who have suffered from one or more of these tragic illnesses.

But what about you? Is there anything you can do to reduce the risk of your being stricken by one of these present-day killers? Recent research indicates that you can. By making a few simple changes in your lifestyle, you can lessen the risk of many common diseases by as much as fifty percent.

Your chances of remaining healthy are greatly increased if you eliminate cigarettes, alcohol, and caffeine. At the same time, you should include daily exercise, adequate water, and sufficient rest in your routine. Most of all, you should change the *way* you eat and *what* you eat.

You may be saying, "Why should I change my way of eating, I'm not sick." But are you physically healthy and robust? Or do you often feel tired, depressed, unmotivated to work, restless, sleepless , and generally unhappy? The remedy for you is probably a balanced diet. I have seen these sluggish feelings disappear when people have changed their eating habits and taken steps to regularly eat adequate amounts of healthful foods.

Maybe your problem is your weight. Can being overweight affect your health? Being 20% overweight is a risk factor in kidney disease, high blood pressure, certain types of cancer, diabetes, gallstones, and heart disease.

Fat Can Be Beautiful

Nobody wants to be fat, but everyone needs some fatty tissue. Fat can be beautiful when it is stored in several strategic spots on our bodies.

Fatty tissue serves as *pads*—cushions on the soles of your feet, on your hands, cheeks, on your "sitters," along your muscles, and many other places. You would be very uncomfortable without these pads of fat. In addition, life would be unbearable if you got the full impact of every sound in your environment. Fat pads serve as shock absorbers over nerve endings to soften loud noises and shrill sounds.

Fatty tissue is also necessary to *hold the internal organs* in place and keep them from sudden injury during accidents. A dear friend of mine was an eternal weight-conscious dieter wanting to stay skinny as a rail. She began suffering severe back pains. Finally, yielding to an appointment with a physician, she found that all of her internal organs had dropped. Their weight was pressing against the nerve center in her lower back. Five weeks and many dollars later, surgery corrected the problem. The surgeon literally tied one organ to another to substitute for what God had planned so perfectly—the use of fatty tissue to support internal organs.

Fat also acts as *an insulator* against excessive loss of body heat. Very thin people suffer more from cold weather than those who have some layers of fat stored under the skin. When you don't or can't eat properly to meet current demands for heat, these storage cells supply fuel (energy). Fat cells provide a place to *store left-over calories* that your body does not need for immediate use.

God knew what He was doing when He gave both men and women some special storage bins for one of the essential nutrients—fat. Fat is beautiful when it fulfills the purposes God intended.

When Fat Is Ugly

Fat can also be ugly—it displeases the Lord, is offensive to others, and threatens our health.

Fat is ugly when it robs us of our physical beauty. That happens when we are more than 10 percent overweight for our height, age, and bone structure. Here's an easy way for you to calcuate your approximate desirable weight. If you are five feet tall, give yourself 100 points; for women, add

5 points, men add 7, for each additional inch of height.

A woman 5'8" tall should weigh about 140 pounds. (100 points for being 5 feet; 8 inches x 5 or 40 points for the height above 5 feet.) If she weighs more than 10% above 140 (154 lbs.) she is considered overweight. If she weighs as much as 168 or more, she is obese.

Fat is ugly when your internal organs are smothered and squeezed into partial functioning. Excess fatty tissue surrounding your heart forces it to pump blood to *miles* of extra blood vessels every five-sixths (5/6) of a second. For every pound of fat, your body forms and must nourish approximately three-fourths (¾) of a mile of extra blood vessels. So twenty-five pounds of excess fat means more than *eighteen miles* of extra blood vessels to be nourished and flushed, every five-sixths (5/6) of a second!

Mortality rises as the degree of obesity increases. The statistics of the Metropolitan Life Insurance Company (USA) have shown that for a man of 45, an increase of 25 pounds over standard weight reduces life expectancy by 25 percent. In other words, he is likely to die at sixty when he might otherwise have lived to seventy-five or more had he not been obese.[1]

Fat is ugly when it complicates the birth of a baby. A pregnant woman's excessive fat can cause the death of either herself or the child. Some obstetricians refuse to take obese pregnant women as patients because they fear being blamed or sued for the tragic situations that often accompany the delivery of babies of obese mothers.

Fat is ugly when it takes your life while you are in surgery. Surgeons will tell you that your chances of surviving a major operation decrease in proportion as your overweight condition increases. Overweight persons are greater surgical risks.

Little Inconveniences

In addition to being ugly, being overweight can also be inconvenient.[2] Here are some definite inconveniences that an overweight person has:

—*Shortness of breath* and a continuous *tired feeling* which does not go away with more food, more rest, more relaxation, or sleep.

—*More strain* in doing routine daily tasks—like housecleaning, grocery shopping, grass cutting, etc.

—*More "blab" days* and *more absenteeism* from paid employment—with a resultant loss of income.

—*Limited productivity* in certain jobs—with an adverse effect on income.

—Abdominal *hernias* and *vericose veins* more frequently than normal weight adults.

—More *infertility* in men and more *menstrual abnormalities* in women.

—More *infections* of the respiratory tract—such as colds.

—Increased rate of *skin problems*—often caused by excessive perspiration in skin folds.

—*Increased risks* during child delivery and surgery.

Recent statistics estimate that approximately 50% of all American men over thirty and 75% of women over forty years of age are overweight. Large percentages are obese, meaning that they are 20% or more above their ideal weight.

Big Problems

There is another long list of physical conditions which are suffered more frequently by overweight and obese persons than by their counterparts of normal weight. These *more serious illnesses* include:

—*Gall Bladder Disease*

It has been reported that obese individuals suffer three times more gallstones than adults of normal weight.

—*Orthopedic Problems*

Common symptoms are pain in the lower back and joint pains—especially of the hips, knees, and ankles.

—*Complications During Pregnancy*

Obese women suffer seven times more toxemia (especially of the kidney) than normal weight women; five times more infection of the urine-collecting part of the kidney, with more maternal deaths.

—*Respiratory Problems*

In addition to drowsiness and lack of oxygen in the blood, the lungs can also lack oxygen. Breathing is often labored and difficult.

—*Liver Dysfunction*

The Bromsulphalein test, which quantitatively evaluates liver function, shows that liver dysfunction is more frequently a problem among the obese than non-obese.[3]

—*Degenerative Arthritis*

The occurrence of arthritis increases with the increase of weight. Degenerative arthritis was observed among 80% of obese patients in one arthritic clinic. Excess weight adds pressure on the joints. The loss of each pound of excess weight may relieve the hip joint of three pounds of pressure.[4]

The Great Jeopardizers

The obese are more prone than persons of normal weight to have cardiovascular disease, diabetes, hypertension, and, perhaps, cancer. Facts you should know about them are as follows:

—*Cardiovascular Disease* (heart, arteries, capillaries, veins)

About one million Americans die of it annually, and the major cause is overweight and obesity.

Weight gains after 25 years proved to be strongly related to *angina pectoris* and sudden death.

The annual death rate from hardening of the

arteries *(artherosclerosis)* and degenerative *heart disease* in the U.S. for men age 50-59 is the *highest* in the world. Incidence of *coronary artery disease* among Americans increased proportionately with degree of overweight.

—*Hypertension* (high blood pressure)

Research shows that it is not uncommon for overweight people to have much *higher blood pressure* rates than people of normal weight.

Mortality ratios increase as the average systolic and diastolic blood pressure rises. Being overweight and obese causes blood pressure to rise.

Circulatory problems of all kinds are aggravated. Both an increase of blood volume and blood pressure put a strain on the heart.

—*Diabetes* (insufficient insulin to handle sugars and starches)

Statistics show that diabetes is *four times more common* in obese than in lean adults.

A weight gain often precedes the *onset* of adult diabetes.

Underweight persons who are 50 years old or more rarely have diabetes. Contrarily, 80% of *elderly diabetics* are overweight.

The Diabetic Syndrome

Mortality among obese diabetics is four times greater than for the diabetic of normal weight.

According to Dr. Stephen Podolsky, diabetes mellitus is now the third leading cause of death in the United States, accounting for 300,000 lives each year. Only cardiovascular diseases and cancer are responsible for more deaths. If the present trend continues, by 1990 there will be twenty million Americans with diabetes—twice as many as in 1975.

There are two kinds of diabetes: one develops in youth, called *juvenile-onset;* the other develops in later life and is called *maturity-onset.*

Juvenile-onset diabetes is caused by a failure of the body to produce insulin which is needed for the metabolism of carbohydrates (starches and sugars). In *maturity-onset diabetes,* the body cells have an inability to respond normally to insulin. In both types, blood sugar fails to penetrate body cells and they become deprived of vital energy. It is like a "water, water everywhere and not a drop to drink" situation!

For maturity-onset diabetes, lowering body weight to normal and keeping it there eliminates the condition in many cases. Juvenile-onset diabetes, contrarily, is not usually reversible.

A woman I know (who is much overweight for her height and frame) began to have the symptoms of frequent urination, insatiable thirst, dizziness, and headaches. When she went to her physician for an examination, he diagnosed her condition as diabetes (too much sugar in the blood). She was put on a strict diet, with injections of insulin every morning. All sweets were strictly forbidden. The doctor made this very, very plain.

As a lover of sweets all her life, she thought that a little piece of candy wouldn't hurt. She bought her favorite kind, chocolate kisses, and put them in a secret place upstairs in her bedroom. No one knew, she thought; it was a foolproof scheme.

But after supper one night she left the family circle in the living room and tiptoed up to her room to secretly have a piece of her chocolate candy. One piece didn't quite do it. So she had one more. Those two didn't quite satisfy her either. Unable to stop, she ate herself into a diabetic coma!

The panic and confusion that followed sent a shock wave throughout the household and neighborhood. It was quite a spectacle when the fire department arrived and carried her off to the hospital. About $100 and a day later, she was back home feeling guilty and embarrassed for having been so foolish.

Principles To Lose By

Are you one of the 80 million Americans who are overweight? If you've decided that you need to lose those excess pounds, here are a few basic principles for you to follow:

1. *Decrease* your intake of:
   —meat (beef, lamb, pork & pork products)
   —fat (fat meat, fried foods, butter, oil, etc.)
   —sugars (sweets, candy, refined sugars, etc.)

—white-flour baked goods (bread, cakes, doughnuts, etc.)
—total calories (from all food groups)
2. *Increase* your intake of:
   —fresh or frozen vegetables (plain with no butter or sauce)
   —fresh fruits and unsweetened fruit juices
   —lowfat milk (and lowfat milk products)
   —baked or broiled fish and poultry (without butter or skin)
   —whole grain products (bread, cereal, pasta)

This simple plan will help you lose weight safely and will bring about permanent change in your eating habits.

Cancer—You Can Prevent It

There has been much research into the possible relationship between our diets and cancer. Through this research, it has been suggested that high consumption of animal protein, low consumption of fiber, and a high consumption of fat may be linked to *colon cancer*.[5] The more economically developed a society is, the greater the incidence of colon cancer. [6] The high incidence of *breast cancer* among North American and western European women and among immigrants adopting a *high-fat* Western diet points to a possible relationship between high-fat intake and breast cancer.[7]

Experimentally, obesity is also linked with cancer. Obese mice with *high-fat* consumption tend to have a higher *tumor* incidence than normal animals.[8] Animal obesity plays a major role in increasing the risk of cancer of the endometrium and kidney.

The consumption of excessive beer, alcohol, red meats, caffeine, fats, and sugar with low intakes of vitamin C and A have all been cited as related to high cancer incidence.

The American Medical Association has suggested that vitamin A foods (like carrots, sweet potatoes, squash, and dark green, leafy vegetables) and vegetables of the cruciferous family (like cauliflower, brussel sprouts, broccoli, cabbage) appear to be linked to a lower incidence of several kinds of cancer.

The Committee on Diet, Nutrition and Cancer of the National Research Council suggests that we avoid foods that are salt-cured, pickled, smoked, or contain the additives *nitrate* and *nitrite*.

The National Cancer Institute offers a 5-point recommendation concerning diet in the *prevention of cancer*.[9]

1. Eat less fat.
2. Maintain body weight.
3. Eat more dietary fiber.
4. Avoid consuming too many or too few vitamins and minerals.
5. Drink alcohol in moderation.

Dangerous Additives

You would be wise to cut down on foods containing many artificial additives and preservatives. Some dietitians and physicians consider certain chemicals to be dangerous to health when ingested even in small quantities. The list includes: BHA and BHT, caffeine, carrageenan, modified food starch, MSG, nitrites, propylene glycol alginate, red dye 40, saccharin, and sodium erythrobate.

Dr.'s Agatha and Calvin Thrash list the foods containing the *twenty worst additives:*

"Cakes, crackers, pies, and doughnuts contain 11 of the 20 worst ingredients.

"Colas, soft drinks, punches, and powdered drink mixes contain 9 of the 20.

"Pizzas, gelatin, pudding desserts, beer, ice cream, and ice milk contain 6 of the 20.

"Vegetable sauces contain 5; broths and salad dressings contain 4 of the 20 worst ingredients."[10]

Caffeine can also cause health problems. It continues to be reported as a factor associated with high blood cholesterol levels (and heart disease) and with low levels of HDL-cholesterol (the beneficial, heart-protecting form of cholesterol).

Peptic ulcers, diabetes, and hypoglycemia are also adversely affected by caffeine. Recently, some researchers have reported that caffeine causes an alteration in the chromosomes in the nuclei of cells and may be linked to cancer.

How can you tell if you are drinking too much coffee? Give it up for 2-3 days and see if you experience: tiredness, anxiety, insomnia, racing of the heart, finger tremor, imperfect balance, or a sense of dread. If you do, you are using caffeine as a *drug*.

According to one doctor, "If a person regularly drinks one to five cups of coffee a day, his risk of having a heart attack is 60% higher than if he drinks none. If he drinks six or more cups a day, his risk is 120% higher! Caffeine raises blood pressure, causes the heart to race or have extra beats, and interferes with sleep."[11]

We must remember that coffee is not our only source of caffeine. It may not even be the major source! Cola-type drinks, tea, chocolate, cocoa, and medicines are also major sources, as indicated in the following list.[12]

Cocoa Cola	6 oz. bottle	40 mg.	caffeine
Coffee	6 oz.	120 mg.	"
Dr. Pepper	6 oz.	38 mg.	"
Pepsi Cola	6 oz.	36 mg.	"
Tea	6 oz.	100 mg.	"
Decaffeinated Coffee	6 oz.	18 mg.	"

The pharmacological, or drug effect, of caffeine is achieved when we take 60-100 milligrams into our bodies.

Three Life-Changing Diets

The way you eat affects the condition of your health. By making a few changes in your diet you can bring some diseases and unhealthy conditions under control.

1. *Lower your blood pressure by the way you eat.*

There is a significant relationship between the amount of salt consumed and our blood pressure. Eating highly salted foods, especially snack foods, makes salt consumption excessively high. It has been estimated that many Americans eat about *ten times* more salt than is required for good health. The amount recommended is 7/8 of a teaspoon daily!

A low-sodium (salt) diet is an excellent way to help keep your blood pressure under control. Reducing your intake of sugar and white flour foods will also help lower blood pressure.[13] The ups and downs in blood glucose will moderate, and exaggerated fluctuations in personality characteristics (ranging from hyperactive to catatonic) will decrease.

People with an inadequate intake of *potassium* often develop hypertension. This problem can be deferred by eating foods rich in potassium like: peanuts, peas, dark green, leafy vegetables, dates, bananas, cantaloupe, dried beans, and potatoes. Meats are also a good source of potassium.

Other measures that are effective in lowering blood pressure are: exercising daily, lowering weight to normal, and eliminating smoking.

2. *A low-fat diet can clear clogged arteries and help heal victims of heart attacks and strokes.*

Research from many sources conclude that arteriosclerosis can be reversed when the fat calories in the diet are lowered to 10% of our total calorie intake. That would mean giving up *all* fried foods, butter, milk, cheese, salad dressings, ice cream, hamburger, potato chips, pork, or "extra-crispy" fried chicken (which equals 18 pats of butter in a half-chicken serving!).

If you've never had a heart attack or stroke, you can decrease your chances of having one by reducing your fat intake to 25-30% of your total calories.

3. *Some digestive problems can be corrected with proper eating habits.*

It takes the stomach *four hours* to empty an average meal. This means that snacking between meals adds food to an already working stomach and increases the emptying time—sometimes to as much as *nine hours.* In addition, the fermentation which is created in the stomach can be detrimental to your mind, body, and emotions. It is recommended that *five hours* be allowed to lapse between the end of one meal and the next time you eat.

Some people nibble and snack all day instead of eating proper meals. This can be very harmful to your body because it causes poor absorbtion of nutrients and reduces the amount of protein available for the body to use.[14]

Here are seven simple dietary guidelines that can change your life and improve your health.[15]

The way you eat definitely affects your health— either positively or negatively. If you want to live without feeling sick and tired, your diet will have to change. Our bodies have natural healing mechanisms that respond to proper nutrients. If you put the right foods in, you'll get a healthy body in return.

1 Eat a Variety of Foods

2 Maintain Ideal Weight

3 Avoid Too Much Fat, Saturated Fat, and Cholesterol

4 Eat Foods with Adequate Starch and Fiber

5 Avoid Too Much Sugar

6 Avoid Too Much Sodium

7 If You Drink Alcohol, Do So in Moderation.

Chapter Seven

YOU AND YOUR WEIGHT

Can being overweight affect your lifestyle and the way you live?

Studies show that more non-obese than obese high school graduates go on to college. In most careers, people without a college education cannot secure and remain in the same kinds of jobs as those with a college education. So a person's earning power for his whole life could be adversely affected by his overweight or obese conditions.

Some employers have a policy of not hiring overweight people. Law enforcement, home economics, dietetics, commercial airlines, and fashion merchandising are some careers that often enforce this policy.

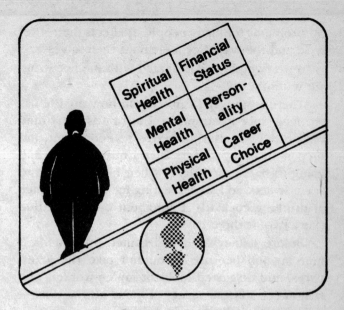

The editor for a newsletter published by Weight Watchers, Inc. conducted a study to determine how fat people are succeeding in the job market. Her conclusion was that they would be more successful if they lost weight. Limited job opportunities, failure to secure jobs, fear of applying for a promotion or a new position are part of the lifestyle of some obese people. This adds up to salary not earned, forfeited benefits, and a loss of professional prestige.

Self-Esteem And Your Weight

Being overweight causes social and psychological problems for many people. It affects their life-style and the way they feel about themselves.

An overweight friend shared with me her struggle with obesity.

"There is no way I can tell you how my life has changed since I became fat. Until I was thirty-nine years old, I was slim, attractive, self-confident, and successful in my career. Then I quit drinking and going to bars every night. When I did, I began to crave sweets. So I started eating ice cream in place of drinking cocktails. I ate about one-half gallon every two or three days.

"Before I knew it, I had gained 59 pounds. I quit my job because I couldn't take the jokes, stares, and disgusted looks of my co-workers and customers. I began to stay at home all the time—not wanting to be seen in public.

"When I went shopping for necessities, I used to look behind me to see if people were making fun of me. Sometimes they were! This pushed my hatred of being fat even more deeply into my subconscious mind. It was terrible!

"Even my own family put me through some humiliating experiences. My children tried to be kind, but they often remarked, 'Mother, you sure are fat. Can't you stop eating so much?' My husband is the only one who doesn't mention my weight. But even if he doesn't, I know what he is thinking and I am ashamed for him to see me undressed.

"All of these tortures are only part of my problem. I have tried every diet I ever heard about. At various times in the past twenty years, I have joined weight-loss programs, some costing nearly $200 a month. I spent thousands of dollars on doctors, chiropractors, and the medicines they recommended. Nothing has resulted in successful, sustained weight loss.

"Every aspect of my life has changed since I gained weight. I won't apply for a job even though I could help my husband with our children's college expenses. But I can't face being rejected. I know no one would hire me.

"I've even stopped going to church. I've dropped out of everything I used to enjoy, and I just sit at home and watch TV. I'm not physically able to even push a vacuum cleaner. At the slightest amount of physical labor, I get short of breath. My doctor told me I have high blood pressure and diabetes. And there seems to be no solution."

Her interview ended with a question: "Do you have any suggestions for me?" I certainly did!

How To Go On A Diet

Every year people in the U.S. spend millions of dollars trying to find a fast and easy way to lose the weight they put on over a period of years. The costs of obesity range from doctors visits to health spas with millions spent on appetite depressants and low-calorie soda pop. Yet many people regain the weight they lose.

One of the most effective weight-loss programs

is still good old-fashioned dieting. The first step to successful dieting is to realize you must make a change in the way you eat—not a temporary fling but a permanent change. Long-term results should be your motivation.

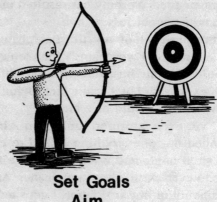

Set Goals
Aim
Fire!

Next, set your goals. Decide how much you want to lose and how long you think it will take you. Lose weight slowly—never more than two pounds each week. This will give you time to develop good eating habits that will last the rest of your life.

Here are some guidelines to use in selecting a good diet program:

1. Do not choose a diet that supplies less than *800-1000 calories* a day. Your body needs maintaining, even while you are losing weight.

2. Do not use a *liquid diet* as your only source of

nutrients. Taking only liquids can cause the muscles of your intestines to get sluggish from underactivity. Colon problems can result when you resume normal eating. A high-protein liquid diet can cause a nutritional imbalance in the body. This can prevent the heart from being able to receive proper electrical impulses. The result can be sudden death.

3. Choose a diet that includes an *exercise program*. Physical exercise will help strengthen your muscles and prevent flabby and sagging skin that makes you look older.

4. Choose a diet that includes all of the *basic food groups*—fruits, vegetables, cereals, legumes, milk products, and meat. Your diet should be balanced—not "high" in anything.

5. Do not ignore your own *special health needs*. Check with your doctors before beginning the diet to make sure it does not conflict with any medications or health problems you may have.

The More You Eat, The More You Want

Have you ever heard of a person who wagered a bet that he could eat more pie or more pancakes than anyone in their city or town? Then everyone goes to the civic center or the fairgrounds to watch the contestants stuff themselves.

The Guinness Book of World Records records all kinds of death-defying statistics:

Ice cream—3 pounds (unmelted) eaten in 90 seconds.

Pancakes—62 (each 6" in diameter, buttered and with syrup) consumed in 6 minutes, 68.5 seconds.[1]

It amazes me that these contestants didn't drop dead on the spot!

When we eat large amounts of concentrated sweet foods (the sugars and starches in the form of candies, baked desserts, ice cream, pancakes with syrup, biscuits with honey) the body is put under great stress. It gears up for this emergency situation in miraculous ways.

Let's say you eat a candy bar. The candy bar contains a concentrated solution of sugar that actually causes the lining of the stomach to hurt. The nerves in the stomach lining send a message to the brain, "Hey, I have been flooded with a super-saturated solution of sugar, and it is painful. Do me a favor; make this person thirsty. Tell him to take a drink of water so the sugar will be diluted. That will help a little bit. Then send a message to the pancreas, and tell it to speed up the production of insulin to handle all this sugar."

The brain does exactly what the messages coming into it say should be done. It tells you to get a drink, and it speaks plainly to the pancreas, which responds immediately. More insulin comes quickly flowing in.

The pancreas speeds up, working faster and faster as it works harder and harder. Before long it has enabled the body to handle the flood of sugar. Some has been stored in the liver, some in the muscles, some converted to fat, and some used for energy.

When the supply of sugar is accommodated, the pancreas sends out an S.O.S. to the brain. It says, "Hey! Go tell my boss to go to the refrigerator and eat some more food. I'm geared up for work, and it takes me awhile to slow down. If I send more insulin into his stomach, he will black out in an insulin shock." This condition scares everybody. The victim looks and acts as if he's going to die, and some do.

If you eat sweets right before you go to bed, you may awaken in the middle of the night with a strong urge to get something more to eat. Promise yourself that you will learn not to flood your body with concentrated sweets, especially on an empty stomach or before going to bed at night.

What's So Bad About Sugar?

Sugar and sweet foods are such a part of our lives that it's hard to believe they could be all that bad for us. Americans grow up with decorated cakes on birthdays, cookies at Christmas, candy on Valentine's Day, and dessert after supper. How could something that centers around so many fond memories be so sinister? Let's look at some of the health problems created by this innocent-looking substance.

1. Sugar *adds only calories* and pounds to our bodies. It contains absolutely *no* vitamins, minerals, amino acids, or other nutrients.

2. Excess sugar causes a rise in blood fat. This condition contributes to *high blood pressure* and heart attacks.

3. *Cavities* in our teeth are primarily caused by eating too much sugar. Chewing gum and candy that remain in the mouth for long periods of time bathe the teeth with sugar and create cavities.

4. Sugar causes a rapid rise in blood sugar levels—sometimes causing a person to swing from *hypoglycemia* to diabetes within a one-hour period (or even less). Headaches, fatigue, forgetfulness, irritability, and blurred vision can result.

5. Too much sugar in the diet can trigger the onset of *diabetes* in individuals with an inherited weakness toward this disease. It causes the arteries to narrow so that the blood flow is hindered. This brings on premature aging and affects the eyes and kidneys. (Diabetes is the number one cause of new cases of blindness in the U.S.) People with diabetes often suffer disabling complications and have a shortened life span.

6. Sugar decreases the body's ability to destroy bacteria and fight infection. When we eat as much as 24 teaspoons of sugar in a short time, the ability of the white blood cells to destroy bacteria is decreased by about 92%. Our immune system is impaired, and we become easy prey to *infections* of all kinds. (The average American eats 42 teaspoons of sugar every day—in some form or another.)

Do we need *any* sugar in our diets? No! We do

not need any *simple* sugars like: Cane sugar, brown sugar, honey, molasses, corn syrup, etc. If we eat fruits and complex carbohydrate foods (beans, peas, nuts, seeds, vegetables, whole grain breads, and cereals), we get more than enough sugar in our diets.

In other countries where people eat 80% of their total diet in the form of complex carbohydrates, they have virtually no tooth decay, no heart attacks, no cancer, no obesity, and no arthritis. Is it worth giving up sugar and sweets to have the benefit of good health and a productive life?

The Impulsive Eater

Many of the super-sweet foods that we enjoy are eaten on impulse. We usually give little thought at the time to what all that sugar will do to our bodies and minds.

Have you ever been walking down the street and passed a doughnut shop? The odor drifting into the street announces a fresh batch of "so-fats." Not having had a fresh doughnut for a few days (hopefully weeks) you decide to rest your tired feet and have a cup of coffee and a doughnut.

Your feet weren't really *that* tired, and heaven knows you didn't need the food. You had left the breakfast table only two hours before, but the enticement of that delicious odor was more than you could resist. Impulsively you made the choice to overeat.

Maybe you can't identify with yielding to the

smells of a doughnut shop. But that doesn't mean you aren't an impulsive overeater. What about the 33 flavors at the ice cream store, caramel-covered popcorn at the movies, or a candy bar at the check-out counter? What about the small mint at the cash register of your favorite restaurant? After all, it contains from 50 to 100 calories, and you just finished a big meal before you paid your bill!

The Frustrated Eater

We all eat more than we should from time to time, but some people habitually overeat. Their reasons for overeating are often emotional or psychological. They may feel unloved, unwanted, unneeded, lonely, disappointed, guilty, or fearful. Or they may be overworked, pressured, anxious, and worried.

One of my secretaries whose husband works at night often finds herself feeling restless and afraid because she's alone. Her emotions sometimes get the best of her, and she often finds herself standing in front of the refrigerator. Before she realizes what she's doing, she eats everything in sight— consuming thousands of calories without even thinking.

Work or academic situations can also produce feelings of frustration. You may be working on an assignment or a project and come to a point where you don't know what to do next. Before you know what is happening, you head for the coffee pot and all the goodies that surround it—the cookie jar, the doughnut box, or the leftover birthday cake. Trying to soothe your shattered nerves, you swallow 300, 400, 500 calories in a few minutes and end up feeling worse instead of better. The sugar in your system only increases your feeling of frustration and confusion. In addition, the unnecessary caffeine jangles rather than soothes your frazzeled nerves.

Your frustration may be covered up, but the extra pounds that cling to your waist and double chin can't be disguised.

Overworking Your Heart

In the gospel of Luke, Jesus gives us a very serious warning: "Take heed to yourselves, lest at any time your hearts be overcharged with surfeiting (overeating) and drunkenness, and cares of this life, and so that day comes upon you unawares" (21:34).

"Lest your hearts be overcharged." It could have two meanings—a spiritual and physical one. When the heart becomes encased in a mass of fat, it becomes heavy and unable to perform its duties effectively and efficiently. Fatty deposits around the heart increase its workload. If you are 20 or 50 or 70 pounds overweight, your heart has to service an equivalent number of *miles* of extra blood vessels. Your heart can't take such stress forever. That kind of heaviness of the heart will shorten your life, as the vital statistics prove.

Another definition of the overcharged heart

requires spiritual interpretation. Deuteronomy 32:15 says that when the Israelites became overfed, yes, fat and bloated, they forgot their God. "They shrugged away the Rock of their salvation" (*TLB*).

If the Israelites were harmed spiritually by their bodily fatness, could it be the same with us today?

The Consequences

Fatness has detrimental effects on our spirituality. In Deuteronomy 31:19-21, God spoke to Moses and said, "Now write down the words of this song, and teach it to the people of Israel *as my warning to them*. When I have brought them into the land. . .'flowing with milk and honey'— and when they have become fat and prosperous, and worship other gods [like food and drink] and despise me and break my contract, and great disasters come upon them, then this song will remind them of the reason of their woes. (For this song will live from generation to generation)" (*TLB*).

An obese friend told me that as long as you bless your food before you eat it, you do not have to worry about your weight; God will keep you in good health. A few months later, however, this person had an attack with all the symptoms of a slight stroke. It's true that we reap what we sow, even in the area of overeating or overdrinking.

Letting our bodies get fat is detrimental to our spiritual and physical health. We should not permit an overweight or obese condition to persist in our lives because it is not pleasing to our God. If we fail to take heed we may, in the end, feel like Cain when he said, "My punishment is greater than I can bear" (Genesis 4:13). Our punishment could easily be premature death. That *is* more than we can bear!

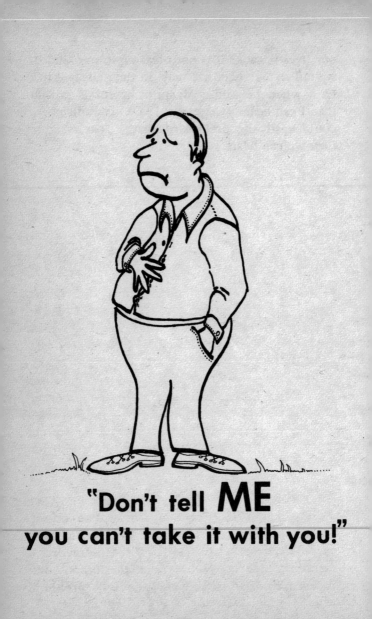

"Don't tell **ME**
you can't take it with you!"

Chapter Eight

THE ANSWER YOU'VE BEEN LOOKING FOR

What is the solution to overeating and obesity? Americans have tried drug therapy, hypnosis, fat removal by surgery, over-the-counter aids (appetite depressants, etc.), diets of many kinds, group therapy, punishment and reward techniques, even prayer and fasting. But few have experienced lasting results.

Diet researchers have come to one conclusion: *there is no completely successful method of dieting that works for everyone over a sustained period of time.* Most adults who lose weight return to their original overweight condition within two years after they stop dieting. That is definitely not success!

I have known dozens of individuals who have struggled with their own methods of diet control. Many have sought trained medical advice and been given "speed-em-uppers," "slow-em-downers," "hold-the-liners," and "knock-em-outers." But drugs have not solved their weight problem.

Instead, they got hooked, became nervous, and had personality changes.

Drugs and other weight-loss techniques often postpone or prevent our finding the permanent solution to diet problems.

Why Diets Fail

When we begin a diet, we usually have something motivating us to lose weight. It may be to:
—look better in a swim suit
—become more physically attractive
—get a new job
—overcome a health problem
—attract the opposite sex
—become more self-confident

All of these reasons are related to what we think, feel, and want. They all revolve around our soulish desires.

People who lose weight for these reasons don't keep it off. In more than 90% of the cases, most people who diet regain the weight they have lost. In fact, many regain *more* than their original weight.

The problem with this kind of motivation is that it isn't good enough. Motivation to change must come from a higher and stronger source than ourselves. It must come from our *spirit*—from our desire to be in line with the will of God for our lives.

The word *diet* comes from the Greek word meaning "manner of living." Our diets are a way of life. The way we eat and the reasons we diet tell a lot about the spiritual condition of our lives.

Eating is not just a physical matter. For some it is an emotional outlet. For others it is a spiritual problem that requires spiritual answers. Controlling your appetite and forming good eating patterns requires spiritual understanding and spiritual methods.

Evaluate Yourself

What must God think when He looks at our country? There are an estimated 80 million Americans who are overweight or obese. That's one out of every four adults! Are you one of them?

Here's a test to help you evaluate your eating habits. You can determine for yourself if your ways line up with God's ways.

Circle true or false to answer each statement.

1. I do everything, even my eating and drinking, to bring glory to the Lord. (See 1 Corinthians 10:31.) *true false*
2. My highest goal is to preserve my body so that God can use me for years of productive work. *true false*
3. God does not mean for me to eat more food than I need: so I don't. (See 1 Corinthians 6:13.) *true false*
4. My weight is normal for my sex, height, age, and activity level. *true false*
5. I do not spend money for foodstuffs that are

not nutritious. (See Isaiah 55:2,3.) *true false*

6. I do not buy foods with empty calories like sweets, soft drinks, candy, alcohol, etc. *true false*

7. As a form of discipline, I regularly deny myself food. (See 1 Corinthians 9:27.) *true false*

8. I am a good example to others in my eating and drinking habits. (See Titus 2:7.) *true false*

9. I seldom stuff myself at a meal because God's Word warns me against it. (See Proverbs 23:1.) *true false*

10. I keep my weight under control because I do not want to harm my body, which is God's home. (See 1 Corinthians 3:16,17.) *true false*

How well did you do on this test? If you are walking in God's ways, then all your answers are true. If you can't answer true to every statement, then the Lord is ready to help you change.

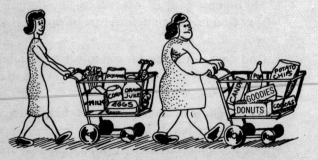

'By their market baskets, ye shall know them.'

Proverbs 3:6 says, "In everything you do, put God first, and he will direct you and crown your efforts with success" (*TLB*).

Your True Nature

Learning to eat properly, like learning to control all other innate appetites within us, is a *spiritual* matter. It requires, therefore, the application of spiritual truths and the use of spiritual weapons. God *is,* and He is *one deity* in three Persons—Father, Son, and Holy Spirit. The Triune God created *triune man.* He made us and said that He was pleased with His creation.

God has a perfect plan for everyone. To understand God's perfect plan for our lives, we need to understand how He said we were made to function. Experience has shown that neither scientists nor philosophers have been able to truly understand the nature of man. They probably never will if they continue to use only the scientific method, inference, or reason.

The Bible teaches that man is *one* person but three elements—spirit, soul, and body. (See 1 Thessalonians 5:23.) Scripture further teaches that we are made in "the image and likeness of God" (Genesis 1:27).

How You Make Decisions

God created our bodies with *five senses* to use in the decision-making process. They help us distinguish between pleasant and unpleasant experiences, between pleasure and pain. Our taste buds function from birth, and as children we learn to like certain tastes and dislike others.

In the realm of touch, some objects feel soft and pleasurable while others are sharp, prickly, and uncomfortable. Our ears and nervous system find certain levels of sound soothing; others can be painful. Odors that we smell and sights that we see bring happy or unhappy responses.

All of these responses are recorded in the brain, which continually gathers information and stores it for later use. From this collection of stored facts, we form our beliefs and make our daily decisions.

Man became a living soul when God formed him out of the dust of the ground and breathed into his nostrils the breath of life. (See Genesis 2:7.) The soul is composed of three parts—the mind (intellect), the emotions, and the will. The soul is housed in the body, and it is the *control center* over our body.

The soul is the seat of the decision-making powers. Our *will* cooperates with our *mind* and our *emotions* to say in regard to a matter, "I am or I am not;" "I will or I will not;" "I can or I cannot."

The soul controls our *beliefs*. Behavioral psychologists have shown conclusively that we behave in terms of our beliefs. Our beliefs are formed, modified, and solidified as a result of the cooperative working of our mind, our emotions, and our will—the threefold nature of the soul. Hence, the soul controls our behavior.

More Than Willpower

Most dieters try to use *willpower* to control overeating. I know because I've tried it myself.

My mother was a marvelous cook, and often before visiting her I would decide I was not going to break my dietary routine. I would try to envisage myself refusing all the freshly baked pies, cookies, muffins, and biscuits laden with homemade butter and honey. In my mind, I repeated over and over, "I will not overeat."

As soon as I stepped inside the house I would smell a freshly baked pie. My *mind* told me, "Yum! You've had that before." My *emotions* said, "You like that kind of pie, and your mother made it just for you." My *will* would try to respond with, "I shouldn't eat any."

My willpower usually worked until I sat down at the table with my mother. Then she would say, "Come on and help me finish this up. It will never be better than now!" "Have another piece; you eat like a mouse." "You can diet when you get back home; enjoy yourself while you're here on vacation."

That's when I discovered that willpower is not enough. It takes more than willpower to stop that kind of temptation. It takes *won't power* that comes only from the power of the spirit within us.

Our spirit has to convince and persuade our

soul to make the right decisions. Our soul must be brought under the control of our spirit. But our spirit functions only to the extent and in the way that the soul decides.

Controlling Your Appetite

What does the Bible say about man's spirit? In the first place, it tells us that we have one! "But there is a spirit in man: and the inspiration of the Almighty giveth them understanding" (Job 32:8).

Education does not make a man wise. Instead, it is the *spirit* in a man, the breath of the Almighty, that makes him intelligent. God's Spirit operating on the spirit of man brings true understanding. *True wisdom* and absolute knowledge are spiritual, not soulish in nature. Wisdom is not related to our mental ability (our intelligence) or our level of education. The two are quite different.

The Bible also talks about a wisdom that does not come from God. Instead, it is earthly, sensual, and devilish. (See James 3:15.) The Bible contrasts this with another kind of wisdom. "But the wisdom that is *from above* is first pure, then peaceable, gentle, and easy to be intreated, full of mercy and good fruits, without partiality, and without hypocrisy" (verse 17). How do we get this kind of wisdom from above?

According to the words of Jesus, He alone is the one doorway into the hidden wisdom of God. No man can have access to the wisdom that comes from above unless he comes to the Father through

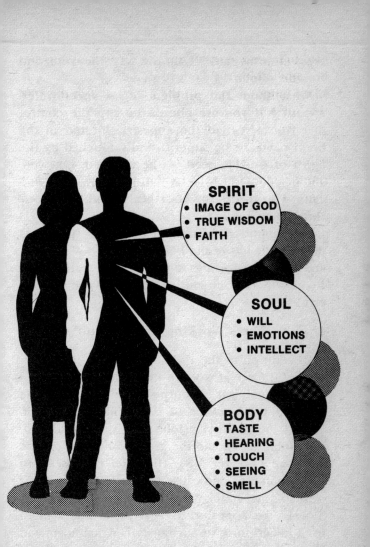

SPIRIT
- IMAGE OF GOD
- TRUE WISDOM
- FAITH

SOUL
- WILL
- EMOTIONS
- INTELLECT

BODY
- TASTE
- HEARING
- TOUCH
- SEEING
- SMELL

the Son. Jesus said, "I am the way, the truth, and the life" (John 14:6).

What about the problem of an uncontrolled appetite? If you are obese, the appetite control mechanism, called the appestat, located in the brain needs to be supernaturally touched by the Spirit of God. It needs to be changed, renewed, and healed. Otherwise, it will go its own way and cause you to destroy your health and your body through overeating.

In the initial creation of man, our spirit was made in the image and likeness of God. Why, then, are we such weaklings in the spiritual realm of our lives? Why has our soulish realm become so powerful?

Who's Working Against You?

In addition to the Holy Spirit, there is another powerful force at work in the world. This force is also spiritual, but his purposes are evil. His name is Satan the *accuser* of the saints (Revelation 12:10) the *destroyer* (John 10:10), the *father of lies* (John 8:44), and the grand *adversary* of God and man (1 Peter 5:8). His chief purpose is to prey upon men and cause them to sin.

Satan's first attack on man is recorded in Genesis 3 when he appeared as a *serpent*—the symbol used in Scripture to portray evil. When Adam and Eve yielded to Satan's temptations, the image of God in man was damaged.

The Bible makes it clear that Adam's fall was the

134

work of an evil spiritual force outside of himself. Our "falls" are often the result of wrong thinking, wrong feeling, and wrong behaving prompted by an evil force working against us. It is the devil's work to pervert and destroy the likeness of God in us. Once we accept and understand this concept, we can begin to make progress toward becoming *whole* persons who live *holy* lives!

The evil force of Satan works against the teaching of Christ—even in a matter as simple as our eating and drinking. Satan tries to deceive us into believing that these ordinary daily functions are not spiritual matters.

God provided the Holy Spirit to reveal Himself to men—to teach spiritual truths and show us how to worship Him. Satan uses false prophets and teachers to persuade us to believe false ideas and doctrines. He wants us to worship him—the prince of this world. Satan's main tool in accomplishing this goal is *deception*. Let's look at some of the counterfeit ideas Satan uses to deceive people.

The Education Myth

Many people believe that education will provide the solution to their problems. They think, "If we teach children what is good and bad about dietary habits, our nutrition problems will be solved."

The education received in public schools is almost entirely centered on *human* knowledge.

Judging from the critical problems in our society, this kind of knowledge has *not* been very effective at changing human behavior!

Millions of dollars have been spent on producing educational materials of the highest quality. Billions more have been spent to hire "the experts" to use these teaching tools in the classrooms. Their goal has been either to dissuade young people from using alcohol, drugs, and cigarettes, or to persuade them to eat breakfast and drink milk. But the facts imparted to the mind have not produced change in our children's lives.

If education worked, we would not have obese dietitians, cigarette-smoking doctors, or millions of young drug addicts and alcoholics. Education of *the psyche* is not the answer.

I was impressed by a verse in Proverbs which says, "It is senseless to pay tuition to educate a rebel who has no heart for truth" (Proverbs 17:16 *TLB*). The soul realm, especially the mind, is the home of "the rebel." For change to take place the rebel must humble himself and submit to the Spirit or be doomed!

The Do-It-Yourself Deception

Another popular counterfeit idea is the one that says, "It is absurd to believe in God. Believe in man, instead. Believe in *yourself*. You are big enough, intelligent enough, sufficient enough, talented enough to solve any problem and solve it perfectly. You belong to an enlightened generation who, with the discoveries of science and the practice of psychiatry, have no need for a so-called God."

People who believe in man without the need for God are called *humanists*. There are millions of them in America today. You can hear them everywhere saying, "Do your own thing." "Be your own person." "Make your own rules." "Eat, drink, and be merry for tomorrow may never come. Even if it does. *You* are in full control."

However, very few people can successfully use the *do-it-yourself* plan for getting rid of a perverted habit, regardless of what that habit is. It takes the power of the Holy Spirit working in harmony with the spirit of man for believers to be overcomers.

Is Gluttony A Sin?

Many Christians are deluded about what is and is not *sin*. I define sin as *going away from good, going away from God*.

Most Christians probably think it is a sin to drink whiskey, smoke marijuana, commit adultery, and tell lies. But *gluttony* (defined in the dictionary as one who eats to excess) is not condemned by most churchgoing people. In fact, it is faithfully practiced by them.

The Bible warns us about gluttony. "Be wise and stay in God's paths; don't carouse with drunkards and gluttons, for they are on their way to poverty" (Proverbs 23:21 *TLB*).

"Take the matter of eating. God has given us an appetite for food and stomachs to digest it. But that doesn't mean we should eat more than we need (1 Corinthians 6:13 *TLB*).

These verses make it clear that God is not pleased with those who overeat and feed their flesh. It may be difficult to admit that gluttony is a sin, but it is the first step toward your freedom.

The Bible says, "If we confess our sins, he is faithful and just to forgive us our sins, and to cleanse us from all unrighteousness" (1 John 1:9). Confession brings forgiveness, and forgiveness leads to change and a new way of living.

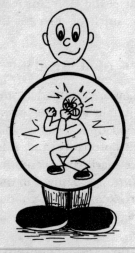

The Battle Within You

Maybe you have confessed your sin of gluttony to God, but you can't seem to stop overeating.

There seems to be something within you that wants to overeat.

Each of us has a natural tendency to indulge ourselves—to follow our whims and urges in search of pleasure and happiness. At the same time, there is a desire within us to obey God and please Him with the way we live.

The apostle Paul struggled with this same inner conflict: "No matter which way I turn I can't make myself do right. I want to but I can't. When I want to do good, I don't; and when I try not to do wrong, I do it anyway" (Romans 7:18,19 *TLB*). This teaching should bring new hope to every Christian who has been unsuccessful in losing weight.

Paul went on to say, "Now if I am doing what I don't want to, it is plain where the trouble is: sin still has me in its evil grasp. . . .I love to do God's will so far as my new nature is concerned, but there is something else deep within me, in my lower nature, that is at war with my mind and wins the fight and makes me a slave to the sin that is still within me. In my mind I want to be God's willing servant but instead I find myself still enslaved to sin" (Romans 7:20-23 *TLB*).

Most of us have felt this way, especially when we are dieting. The battle within us is spiritual in nature—two spirits are at war. The only way to win the battle is to get the Commander-In-Chief on your side. If you ask Jesus to come into your life, He will give you His own spiritual nature.

With Jesus' nature within you, your spirit rises to the top and your body is brought under the control of your spirit. Jesus gives you the power to control your appetite and change your eating habits.

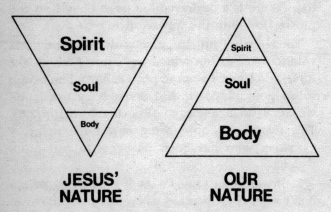

To fight a spiritual battle, you need spiritual help—and Jesus is the answer! Put Him in control of your life.

Chapter Nine

FIGHTING THE WAR AGAINST FAT

You are in a war against fat! If you want to win, you must enlist as a combat soldier. If you don't enlist voluntarily, you may be drafted into the fight by a heart attack, a case of diabetes, high blood pressure, or some other disease caused by being overweight. Or your doctor may force you to enlist in order to save your life.

If you are overweight and past 35 years of age, this is a battle you'll fight for the rest of your life. So sign up and you'll reap all the benefits of a career soldier: a high rank and full retirement. But remember you can't go AWOL. A good soldier reports for duty every day, dressed for battle and ready to fight.

Like all soldiers, you must realize that you can't win the battle alone. You need a leader to guide you and supply you with the necessary equipment. If you are a Christian, your Commander-In-Chief, Jesus Christ, will always be there to boost you on to victory and give you the perfect weapons to use in the battle.

The Overeater's Armor

The apostle Paul tells us what kind of battle we are fighting and how we can win with God's help.

"Put on all of God's armor so that you will be able to stand safe against all strategies and tricks of Satan. For we are not fighting against people made of flesh and blood, but against persons without bodies—the evil rulers of the unseen world, those mighty satanic beings and great evil princes of darkness who rule this world; and against huge numbers of wicked spirits in the spirit world. So use every piece of God's armor to resist the enemy whenever he attacks, and when it is all over, you will be standing up" (Ephesians 6:11-13 *TLB*).

What are the weapons God has given us to use against the enemy? Paul gives us this list: "You will need the strong *belt* of truth and the *breastplate* of God's approval. Wear *shoes* that are able to speed you on as you preach the Good News of peace with God. In every battle you will need faith as your *shield* to stop the fiery arrows aimed at you by Satan. And you will need the *helmet* of salvation and the *sword* of the Spirit—which is the Word of God. *Pray* all the time. Ask God for anything in line with the Holy Spirit's wishes. Plead with Him, reminding Him of your needs" (Ephesians 6:14-18a *TLB*).

FULL ARMOR OF GOD

Ephesians 6:13-17

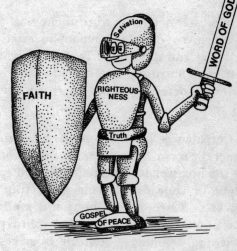

**The Soldier's Garb for ALL Spiritual Battles
Including Overeating!**

Right And True

The Christian soldier's belt is *truth*. It fits around the waist to hold the long tunic in place, and it serves as a holder for the sword. This *belt* gives the warrior freedom to move and freedom to use the hands for battle. Having your hands free increases your fighting power.

The overeater needs the truth about what to eat. This truth gives you the freedom to make right food choices and diet properly. By following the rules of good nutrition, you can win the overeating battle and defeat the problems that accompany being overweight.

The Christian soldier also needs a *breastplate* to protect the torso. The Bible says that *righteousness* is the breastplate. Being morally and spiritually right in your daily living gives you inner power. If you are *right* about the kinds and amounts of food you eat, no one can accuse you of doing wrong (sinning). *Right-ness* makes you impregnable to the enemy and his weapons of warfare. Being right means you have controlled weight.

Defending Yourself

The third piece of the soldier's garb listed by Paul is the *shield*. This piece of armor stops the fiery arrows of the evil one. Those fiery darts are very dangerous weapons. In Paul's time, they were made by covering the end of the dart in cloth, dipping it in pitch, and lighting it with fire. Then it was thrown as a flaming torch at the opposing forces.

Satan will try to oppose you on every side with his fiery darts. They are the temptations that burst into your life without warning: sweets at work, soft drinks on picnics, too much meat at restaurants, fried food at your mother's—the darts fly at us from the most innocent-looking sources.

Satan also uses more subtle darts that sneak around the corner and into our minds. They are thoughts like: "Go ahead and have dessert. You deserve it. One piece won't hurt."

To fight against such fiery temptations, you need a *shield* as your weapon of defense. When used by the Roman soldier, the shield stopped the arrow in its tracks and put out the flame. In spiritual warfare, you can use the shield of faith. Your faith in God and His Word will be your shield against the forces of the enemy.

Prepared To Fight

All soldiers wear *shoes* or boots of some kind. In spiritual warfare, shoes represent readiness—being prepared to fight. When you come home from work at night, you take off your shoes and relax. But a soldier has to sleep with his boots on because he never knows when the enemy will attack.

In your fight against fat, you can never let your guard down. It is a continual battle that must be fought every day—even after you have lost weight and stopped dieting.

The next piece of equipment used in the daily fight against sin is the *helmet*. This important head covering represents salvation—deliverance from the power and penalty of sin.

As a helmet protects the head, salvation protects our minds against the power of sin. It keeps us from making foolish decisions or being ignorant of vital information. Knowledge in the head serves as our deliverer from harm and eventual destruction. With experience, knowledge, and information, we can outwit the enemy and overcome his attempts to kill us—regardless of his tricky schemes.

Ancient soldiers were skilled in the art of sword fighting. In Paul's letter, the *sword* represents the Word of God.

You can use God's Word offensively against the enemy by memorizing several Scriptures dealing with gluttony. Quote these verses aloud to the enemy and tell him you will not be defeated. Memorize other verses dealing with self-control and temperance. Quote these to yourself to strengthen your spirit.

Remember, "When the Holy Spirit controls our lives he will produce this kind of fruit in us. . .self-control" (Galatians 5:22,23 *TLB*).

The Power Of Prayer

God has given us many spiritual weapons to use in our battle against fat: truth, righteousness, readiness, the Word of God, faith, and one final weapon—*prayer.*

Paul said, "Pray all the time. Ask God for anything in line with the Holy Spirit's wishes. Plead with him, reminding him of your needs, and keep praying earnestly for all Christians everywhere" (Ephesians 6:18 *TLB*).

Prayer is the most powerful force in the universe. Believing prayer moves the hand of God on our behalf. To be powerful against the enemy, prayer must be: *constant, intense, unselfish,* and *unwavering*—never doubting. This kind of prayer is the strongest weapon of defense against Satan's attacks.

Your Attitude About Eating

Do you love to eat more than any other daily experience in life? Do all your conversations center around food, restaurants, and recipes? Do you hate the thought of limiting the kinds and amounts of food you eat?

The attitude you have about eating can make or break your attempt to lose weight and stay healthy. Why do you eat? Do you eat to satisfy yourself and your appetite? Or do you eat to bring glory to God?

The apostle Paul wrote, "You must do everything for the glory of God, even your eating and drinking" (1 Corinthians 10:31 *TLB*).

What does the word *glorify* mean? The dictionary definition of *glorify* is to "exalt with praise." Other words that will help us understand *glorify* are: to respect, promote, exalt, adore, credit, esteem, elevate, and magnify. To give glory to God means to honor Him more than we honor ourselves.

In our lives we can glorify God, glorify ourselves, glorify others, or glorify the devil. When we overeat, who gets the glory? We must decide to whom we will give glory, even in our eating and drinking.

Does God demand that we glorify Him? According to the Scriptures, He *demands* and *commands* it. God asks for it with authority and also claims it as His right.

"Haven't you yet learned that your body is the home of the Holy Spirit God gave you, and that he lives within you? Your own body does not belong to you. For God has bought you with a great price. So use every part of your body to give glory back to God, because he owns it" (1 Corinthians 6:19,20 *TLB*).

What is your motive in eating? If you choose to glorify God, there will be a tremendous change in the way you eat—and the way you look!

Paul said it this way, "Give your bodies to God. Let them be a living sacrifice, holy—the kind he can accept. When you think of what he has done for you, is this too much to ask? Don't copy the behavior and customs of this world, but be a new and different person with a fresh newness in all you do and think. Then you will learn from your own experience how his ways will really satisfy you" (Romans 12:1,2 *TLB*).

True satisfaction comes from pleasing God in all we do. What better motive can we have for losing weight and being healthy than to glorify God?

Getting Motivated

We all know that overeating does not please God, and it is dangerous to our health. But how do we go about changing our eating habits?

Change is always difficult. We resist, resent, and rebel to one degree or another—especially when it involves something as near and dear to us eating. But change is easier if we are highly motivated.

An athlete disciplines himself to achieve certain goals because of his strong desire to win. What should be the Christian's motivation?

Paul told us why we should discipline and deny ourselves: "To win the contest you must deny yourselves many things that would keep you from doing your best. An athlete goes to all this trouble to win a blue ribbon or a silver cup, but we do it for a heavenly reward that never disappears. . . .Like an athlete I punish my body, treating it roughly, training it to do what it should, not what it wants to" (1 Corinthians 9:25-27 *TLB*).

For a Christian, pleasing God and doing your

best for Him should be adequate motivation for changing your eating habits. Denying yourself a little food each day is cheaper than joining a health spa or buying diet pills. And the permanent weight loss will mean fewer doctor's fees and medical bills. The positive aspects of self-denial far outweigh the negatives. You can't afford to live without the benefits of normal weight and good health.

If you're sick and tired of feeling sick and tired, then it's time to change. And the way to change is self-denial through the power of God's Spirit within you.

The Sure Remedy

The only sure remedy for getting rid of any unwanted habit is to submit your mind, your will, and your emotions to the mind, the will, and the emotions of God through Jesus Christ. If there is another way to solve your problem, science, medicine, psychiatry, and education have not found it!

A person who has not opened his spirit to the Spirit of God is spiritually dead. (See Ephesians 2:1-5.) He is in spiritual darkness, alienated from God. He does not and cannot understand the things of the Kingdom of God because spiritual matters are spiritually discerned. (See 1 Corinthians 2:14.) He may have a very brilliant mind, but that will not help. His spirit must be connected with God's Spirit to get the power he needs to change his behavior.

Jesus said that the Spirit of *truth* could not be received by the world, "because it seeth him not, neither knoweth him." He went on to tell His disciples, "but you know him; for he dwelleth with you, and shall be in you" (John 14:17). He was referring, of course, to the Holy Spirit.

Before the Holy Spirit can deal with our spiritual problems, He has to be welcomed into our hearts. He has to be invited in! When we allow the Spirit of God to work in and through us, our minds are renewed. In fact, the Bible says that we can have the very mind of Christ Himself. (See 1 Corinthians 2:16.)

God is the only source of true wisdom and understanding. Unless He is in control, we will not and cannot make the best decisions for our lives. We need divine illumination to know the truth. Jesus said it is the truth that sets us free. (See John 8:32.)

Do you want to experience the truth? Do you want to be set free from obesity? Then confess your need for *supernatural* help. Ask the Holy Spirit to strengthen your spirit and, with persistence and patience, *you will overcome*.

Chapter Ten

THE SECRET TO PERFECT HEALTH

Just as Ponce de Leon looked in vain for the fountain of youth, people today continue to search for the secret to perfect health. The problem is that most people are looking in the wrong places.

The secret to perfect health goes beyond the physical realms of life. Man is spirit, soul, and body, and these three areas work together to determine our overall state of health. Poor health in any one area affects other realms of our lives.

How does your spiritual condition affect your body's performance? According to physicians and psychiatrists, our spiritual state of health (our mental and emotional condition) is responsible for about 80% or more of our physical sicknesses. Emotional stress can bring on such conditions as migraine headaches, heart trouble, stomach ulcers, high blood pressure, allergies, nervous disorders, and many others. (For more on this subject, read the book *None Of These Diseases* by S.I. McMillen, M.D.)

In the Old Testament, there are both promises

of health and warnings about disease. God has a promise for those who will diligently hearken to the voice of the Lord, do what is right in His sight, give ear to His commandments, and keep all of His statutes. "I will put none of these diseases upon thee. . .for I am the Lord that healeth thee" (Exodus 15:26).

On the contrary, God warns that those who despise His statutes and break His covenant will be afflicted with sickness and plagues of all kinds. (See Deuteronomy 28.) It is clear that a healthy spiritual condition offers a measure of protection against disease.

The Bible says, "A merry heart doeth good like a medicine; but a broken spirit drieth the bones" (Proverbs 17:22).

A Healthy Spirit

Your spirit is the part of you that is like God and makes you desire to know Him. The size or quality of your spirit is not affected by your place of birth, your church affiliation, or your national origin. God gives each person the capability to develop their spirit to do its maximum potential.

People who are spiritually strong and healthy reflect it in their lives. They have an observable radiance on their faces, sparkle in their eyes, and a high level of energy and vitality. Their friendly enthusiasm and free-flowing smile set them apart from the average person.

On the contrary, people who are spiritually

weak show definite symptoms of a low energy level and inability to concentrate on spiritual matters. They are drowsy during church services, sluggish during prayer, and apathetic about Christian work.

These disorders are due to lack of personal Bible study, prayer, and meditation. When these are neglected, sustained interest in spiritual matters declines and spiritual goals are not achieved.

Your spiritual condition, like your physical condition, can gradually be improved when poor habits are reversed and spiritual nourishment is restored.

Your Mind And Emotions

Your soul is composed of your intellect, emotions, and will. Does your spiritual condition affect any of these areas of your life?

Regarding the mind, the Bible says, "For to be carnally minded is death; but to be spiritually minded is life and peace. Because the carnal mind is enmity against God: for it is not subject to the law of God, neither indeed can be" (Romans 8:6,7).

Our minds can either be centered on carnal (worldly, negative) ideas or on spiritual principles. Thoughts of fear, jealousy, anger, or inferiority cause our minds to be confused and negatively productive. This makes us low.achievers and poor performers in our work, our activities, and our relationships.

Long periods of negative thinking can result in personality changes and bring on apathy, loss of willpower, and severe depression. We can become sad, sulking, stubborn, vicious-tongued people who negatively affect those with whom we live and work.

People with poor spiritual habits usually have lost the will to live, the will to get well, the will to work, the will to be generous, the will to get involved, the will to help others, or the will to commit themselves to high ideals and noble purposes in life.

Turning Negatives Into Positives

What can be done to correct a poor mental condition? Negative attitudes can only be changed by spiritual power—the power that God gives us to control our wills. "God hath not given us the spirit of fear; but of power, and of love, and of a sound mind" (2 Timothy 1:7).

When a person meditates on positive thoughts about persons, places, and things, he becomes a positive, spiritually-minded person. Paul wrote, "Fix your thoughts on what is true and good and right. Think about things that are pure and lovely, and dwell on the fine, good things in others. Think about all you can praise God for and be glad about" (Philippians 4:8 *TLB*).

Studying the Word of God on a regular basis will give you plenty of good food for positive thinking.

155

Eliminating fear and worry from our lives also produces a peaceful mental condition. *Prayer* is the secret to true peace. "Don't worry about anything; instead, pray about everything; tell God your needs and don't forget to thank him for his answers. If you do this you will experience God's peace, which is far more wonderful than the human mind can understand. His peace will keep your thoughts and your hearts quiet and at rest as you trust in Christ Jesus" (Philippians 4:6,7 *TLB*).

Our mental performance is greatly affected by our thoughts, and our thoughts are affected by our spiritual habits.

Fat Souls Are Beautiful

There is a kind of fatness that delights the very heart of God. The prophet Isaiah wrote, "Let your soul delight itself in fatness" (Isaiah 55:26). Spiritually we can eat and eat until our minds, emotions, and wills have a high degree of pleasure, joy, and spiritual fatness. Spiritual food not only satisfies us, but it also makes our souls fat. And *fat souls* are beautiful!

While lean bodies result in better health, strength, growth, appearance, and longevity, this truth is reversed in the spiritual realm. *Fat souls* are the ones who are healthy and attractive. When our spirits are full-grown and mature, our souls become fat. Soul fatness brings our behavior in line with the highest standard possible for humans to achieve—*Christlikeness.*

Jesus Christ had qualities of character that set Him apart from His generation. These character qualities were related to the fact that He was God in the flesh; He was nothing but *good*. His constant exhortation to the disciples was that they, too, could have His character qualities if they were willing to confess Him as their Lord and Savior.

Jesus told His disciples, "I am the good shepherd" (John 10:14) and "I am the door: by me if any man enter in, he shall be saved, and shall go in and out, and find pasture" (John 10:9). If you put your trust in Jesus you will find spiritual food to meet your need for spiritual health and growth.

Paul tells us a number of times that when we turn toward God, we begin to take on the same character traits that Jesus exemplified in His earthly life. Certainly Jesus had a spirit that was full of heavenly nourishment.

When we submit our stubborn and prideful wills to God, He takes over. His power comes flooding into us and does its supernatural and superabundant work. "Christ in you" is the great secret to health and success in life. (See Colossians 1:27.)

Delightful Fruit

A healthy, mature Christian produces fruit that is truly pleasing to God. Jesus said, "I appointed you to go and produce lovely fruit always" (John 15:16 *TLB*) What is the difference between the fruit produced by a fat body and that which is produced by a fat soul? The fruit of a *fat body* is often related to sickness, surgery, limitations, injuries, and stumbling blocks.

The fruits of the *fat soul,* on the other hand, are "the fruits of righteousness which are by Jesus Christ, unto the glory and praise of God" (Philippians 1:11). These fruits are love, joy, peace, long-suffering, gentleness, goodness, faith, meekness, temperance. (See Galatians 5:22,23.)

The fruits of the Spirit are perennial in nature and produced in all stages of life. We are told in the Psalms that the godly will flourish like a palm tree, and grow tall as the cedars of Lebanon. "For they are transplanted into the Lord's own garden, and are under his personal care. Even in old age they will still produce fruit and be vital and green. This honors the Lord, and exhibits his faithful care" (Psalm 92:13-15 *TLB*).

Fruit-bearing Christians are a delight to the very heart of God. Jesus said, "You didn't choose me! I chose you! I appointed you to go and produce lovely fruit always" (John 15:16 *TLB*).

If you're sick and tired of feeling sick and tired, God has the answer for you in His Word. The secrets to physical health and spiritual happiness are in the Bible waiting for you to discover. As you let God nourish your spirit and fatten your soul, those sick and tired feelings will become a thing of the past.

Chapter Eleven

LOVE IN THE KITCHEN

One Thanksgiving day my "family" for dinner consisted mainly of students from the Philippines, Pakistan, Greece, Italy, and Ghana. While we were at the table, the conversation turned to the subject of our favorite foods. I asked each guest to tell us their favorite dish prepared by their mother.

One of the young men from the Philippines said his favorite dish was duck soup made from a just-hatched baby duckling. If his description was correct, the soup contained the whole duckling—feathers and all. Even more amazing, during World War II his father sacrificed for him to have a serving of this soup when it cost $40 a bowl in a Manila hotel!

The young man from Ghana said that his favorite dish was a porridge made from a certain kind of worm that lives under the bark of a specific tree. He told how it took his mother and all nine children an entire day to collect enough worms to make one serving of porridge for each family member. Working that hard and that long for a food delicacy for your children certainly qualifies as real love.

Different Kinds Of Love

There are several words to define different kinds of love. *Eros* is the love between a man and a woman and involves sexual passion. The Greek word *storge* is used to describe family affection. *Philia* describes the deepest kind of devotion that exists between a person and his dearest friend. But the word I want to use for love in the kitchen is *agape*.

According to William Barclay, "The real meaning of *agape* is unconquerable benevolence, invincible goodwill. If we regard a person with agape, it means that nothing that person can or will ever do will make us seek anything but his highest good. Though he injure us and hurt us and insult us, we will never feel anything but kindness towards him."[1]

Dr. Barclay goes on to explain that agape is not an emotional love—like the kind we mean when we speak of falling in love with a person. It is of the emotions all right, but it is also of *the will*. It is the power to love even when we do not like a person—the power to do good to a person who is unlovable or even hostile toward us. Agape seeks nothing but the highest good for a person regardless of the circumstances.

This is the precise kind of Christian love that needs to be at work in the kitchen!

Tough Love

The kind of love needed to provide a nutritious diet for a family today is agape love. It takes supernatural strength from God to be unwavering in our nutrition choices. We must determine to make the right decisions in meal planning, grocery buying, and food preparation.

I can think of no better place for agape love to be shown than in the kitchen. But exercising agape love consistently is not an easy matter. This is what I call *tough love*—the power to do what is right regardless of how others criticize or reject it. Once wise decisions are made, we cannot get soft and let our hearts cause us to go against what our heads tell us is best for the health of our family members. As Paul said in Romans 15:1, "We. . .that are strong ought to bear the infirmities of the weak, and not to please ourselves"—even in the matter of preparing family meals.

TV ads manipulate us to make certain choices that we know are not the best for our families. This same pressure comes from magazine articles, newspaper columnists, food manufactures, and other media sources. Sometimes, even our best friends influence us in a negative way.

Easy Love

Fewer and fewer American women seem willing to go the tough love route in preparing meals. They want the quickest meals possible even when they know the nutrient value of many of these foods is questionable. Quick-fix foods are often high in calories, as well as sugar and fat content.

But who can resist using them when they're so much faster and easier to prepare than fresh foods? Who wants to spend hours washing, peeling, and cooking raw vegetables or dried beans?

This is easy love talking: "Fixing *that* is too much trouble, even if it is good for you." "My kids won't eat it so there's no need to serve it." "I don't have time to go to all that fuss and bother." "I know it's not very good for them, but at least they will eat it!"

This kind of attitude is very natural because it is *easy*. It may be painless when you say it, and you may even be applauded as the "nicest" mom in the neighborhood. But someone will have to pay for your laziness—probably your children.

Blame It On The Cook

When easy love is at work in the kitchen—look out! Many traditional ways of cooking create dietary problems rather than prevent them.

Frying foods in deep fat doesn't injure the fat nor the pan you are using in the process. But it can put a burden on the liver, stomach, the intestines, and all digestive juices. It can burden the skin with duties that are sometimes beyond its ability to perform.

Weak fingernails are also an indication that easy love is at work in the kitchen. Gelatin is not the quick cure-all or the long term solution because it doesn't work. There are several amino acids missing in gelatin, and it has an excess of glycine. Only a balanced diet can remedy the problem of split fingernails.

Would you deliberately sprinkle or throw specks of black pepper in your own eyes or those of your children? "Of course not," you say. Did you know that the stomach lining is more sensitive than the eyeball? Too much pepper can be very irritating to the membranes of the stomach. A doctor charged me a horrendous sum of money to give me that piece of advice when a member of my family had a bleeding ulcer. My inattention to good nutrition in the kitchen was making a painful problem even worse.

Peeling. Coring. Trimming. Scrubbing. Dicing. Slicing. Soaking. All simple words to describe destructive processes that have devastating effects on nutrients in foods. Right under the skin of fruits and vegetables is a heavy layer of nutrients containing minerals that regulate body processes. When we are careless in preparing raw foods, this bountiful supply of vitamins and minerals is thrown away along with valuable roughage. It takes *love in the kitchen* to break those old habits and develop new ways of preparing fruits and vegetables for our families.

Corn, potatoes, green beans—the all-star American big three winners at the dining room table! Why? Because our kids like them. So instead of giving our family a wide assortment of vegetables, we sink into the lazy habit of serving one of these three at nearly every meal.

When I was a post-operative patient in a hospital, five of seven straight meals contained either green beans or wax beans. I told the doctor that if he lost my case, he should blame it on the lack of love and good judgment of the hospital kitchen.

Tough Love In The Morning

Serving *breakfast* demands tough love in the kitchen. If your mother or wife forced you to go without food for 16 out of 24 hours, would you think she loved you? I wouldn't! Yet millions of American homemakers act as if breaking the fast before leaving for school or work should be left up to the individual family member—even the tots! Don't fool yourself.

Tough love in the morning makes sure that the human motors leave the house with enough "gas" in their tank to drive all the places they need to go before lunch time! Can you back your car out of the garage and drive to work on an empty gasoline tank? In the same way, you can't leave the house with an empty stomach and not suffer for it later in the morning. You'll run out of energy just when you need it most—during a test at school, at an important meeting with the boss, or while caring for your toddlers at home.

It takes tough love to get everyone up, run them around the block until they are hungry, and then sit patiently with them while they eat a nourishing, well-balanced breakfast. That calls for the stiffest upper lip that a mother can produce! But it is necessary, if you want to give your family an energetic start for a new day.

Some Loving Guidelines

Here are a few dietary guidelines that will help you express tough, agape love in the kitchen:

1. Feed your family a substantial breakfast every day. Serve your smallest meal at night, preferably three or four hours before going to bed.

2. Avoid foods made from refined grains, like white bread, pancakes, doughnuts, etc. Instead, serve whole grain products like wheat, rye, oats, etc. Remember cooked cereals are more nutritious than dry breakfast cereals.

3. Serve more fruits and vegetables, especially raw or steamed, whenever possible and avoid peeling away the outer skins.

4. Serve beef, pork, or lamb only three times a week. Instead use more fish, chicken, cheese, legume, and egg dishes in your weekly menus.

5. In cooking and serving, limit the use of spices that are hot to the tongue like pepper, chili powder, etc.

6. Limit the amount of desserts, cookies, and other sweets served to your children. Instead, give them nuts, seeds, and dried fruits like raisins, apricots, etc.

7. Do not serve beverages with meals because

this delays digestion. Instead, encourage your family to drink lots of water between meals.

8. Remind your family to eat slowly and chew food thoroughly in order to receive the maximum benefit from their food.

9. As much as possible, serve meals at regular hours and avoid snacks between meals.

10. Experiment with more vegetarian dishes that include dried beans and legumes. Try to limit the amount of hamburger you use.

Love From My Kitchen

To help you show love in your kitchen, I have included several recipes that my family enjoys. I have selected non-meat recipes that have been developed for taste, texture, color, and nutrient value. For a few recipes, I have suggested a menu that will enhance the nutritive content of the meal and make it more appealing.

Golden Grain Nuggets

2 C. cooked brown rice	*Combine* all ingredients
3 C. carrots, grated	*Pour* into greased 2 qt.
2 C. sharp cheddar cheese, grated	casserole dish
	Cover
2 eggs, beaten	*Bake* at 375 for 35-40
2 T. onion, chopped	minutes
1½ t. salt	
dash black pepper	*Serves* 7

Menu
Golden Grain Nuggets
Spinach

Fresh or canned tomatoes
Sprig of parsley
Milk

Golden Grain Nuggets are a delicious combination of cheese, and carrots. The 242 calories per serving allow the addition of other items to complete the meal. The protein is adequate for one meal, and the fat content is lower than the fat in a serving of beef. Since we need to increase our intake of complex carbohydrates, the 21 grams in this recipe are important.

To increase the iron content of the meal, a green leafy vegetable such as spinach could be served. Spinach would also contribute a little protein, few calories, some calcium, more Vitamin A, some of the B-vitamins, and complete the vitamin C requirement of the day. By serving a cup of skim or whole milk, 70% of the RDA for vitamin B_2 would be met. A sprig of parsley or canned or fresh tomatoes would add color and taste to a nutritious meal.

Baked Bulgur

2 C. water or stock	Bring liquid to *boil*
1 C. bulgur	*Add* bulgur, *cover*
	Cook 30 minutes on low heat or until liquid is absorbed
1 can cream soup (mushroom or chicken)	*Combine* all ingredients
	Pour into an oiled 1 qt. casserole dish
⅔ C. milk	*Bake* at 375 for 30-40

1 C. cheddar cheese, grated	minutes

½ t. dry mustard

dash black pepper   *Serves* 6-7

Menu

Baked Bulgur

Lima beans or green peas

Tossed salad, including tomato and green pepper

Fruit

Milk

Bulgur is a cracked wheat cereal that has not been widely used in recent years. However, this recipe offers significant amounts of protein, calcium, and phosphorus. It is low in fat, calories, and cost, but it is not high in any one nutrient. Before discarding this dish and reaching for the hamburger, consider the ways a nutritious meal can be built around bulgur.

Legumes, such as lima beans or green peas, are good sources of iron, some B-vitamins, vitamin C, and vitamin A. The protein in the legumes would also complement the protein of the bulgur. A tossed salad with tomato and green pepper would supply more vitamin C and vitamin A. By adding to this basic dish, you can build a low-cost, low-calorie, nutritious luncheon or dinner.

Jamaican Loaf

1 C. cooked soybeans   *Mix* together

1 C. cooked lentils   *Mash* well

1 C. cooked brown rice

1 small can mushrooms, chopped	*Saute* until soft
1 onion, chopped	
1 clove garlic, minced	
2 stalks celery, chopped	
2 T. soy sauce	
1 T. oil	*Combine* all ingredients
	Pour into an oiled loaf pan
¾ C. bean stock	
1 egg, beaten	*Bake* at 350 for 1 hour
2 t. salt	*Serves* 8

Mediterranean Rice

3 T. olive oil	*Saute* in large frypan until soft
1 large onion, chopped	
1 clove garlic, minced	
1 green pepper, chopped	*Add* vegetables and spices
2 stalks celery, chopped	
5 stuffed olives, sliced	*Simmer* 10 minutes
1 large can (28 oz.) tomatoes, chopped	
3 t. salt	
1 t. oregano	
¼ t. basil	
¼ t. tumeric	
2 C. brown rice, uncooked	*Add* remaining ingredients
1 C. cooked garbanzos or green peas	*Cover*
4 C. stock or water	*Cook* 45 minutes on low heat
	Serves 6

Menu	Menu
Jamaican Loaf	Mediterranean Rice
Green or yellow vegetable	Tossed salad
Fresh salad	Fruit
Milk or cheese	

The Jamaican Loaf and Mediterranean Rice differ greatly in calories per serving. In the Jamaican Loaf, the protein, fat, and carbohyrdrates content is lower than in the Mediterranean Rice, and thus fewer calories per serving. In order to build a meal around the Jamaican Loaf, more food items need to be added. The Mediterranean Rice, however, is almost a meal in itself.

A green or yellow vegetable, a fresh salad, a dairy product, such as one cup of skim milk or one ounce of cheese, served with the Jamaican Loaf would make a nutritious meal without overloading on calories. Including low-calorie dishes in the daily eating plan can help control calorie intake without jeopardizing the nutritional quality.

Even though the calories per serving are high in the Mediterranean Rice, it provides excellent amounts of iron, niacin, vitamin C, and significant amounts of the other vitamins and minerals. A tossed salad would add the "crunch" contrast, and a serving of fruit would be ideal to complete a delicious menu.

Baked Broccoli And Cheese Timball

1 10-oz. pkg. frozen   *Cook* and drain; put in 1

broccoli	qt. casserole
¾ C. nonfat dry milk powder	*Mix* all ingredients together
¾ C. Swiss cheese, grated	
2 eggs, beaten	*Pour* mixture over broccoli
2 T. lemon juice	
2 T. butter, melted	*Bake* at 350 for 45 minutes, with a pan of water on bottom rack of oven
⅛ t. black pepper	
½ t. dry mustard	
1¼ C. vegetable stock or water	
	Serves 5

One serving of this recipe provides 17 grams of high-quality protein in addition to being an attractive and delicious dish.

The milk, cheese, and egg (all animal proteins) are complete protein sources which will improve the utilization of the incomplete protein found in the broccoli. This makes the total protein content of this dish excellent, both in quantity and quality.

Meatless Meatballs

½ C. onion, chopped	*Saute* until soft
2 T. butter	
1 C. pecans, finely chopped	*Mix* all ingredients
2 C. bread crumbs, fine	*Add* sauteed onions
¼ C. wheat germ	*Shape* into walnut-size balls (can be refrigerated 24 hours before baking)
2 C. small curd cottage cheese	
2 eggs, beaten	
¼ t. sage	*Bake* on greased cookie

dash black pepper

2 T. soy sauce

sheets at 350 for 30 minutes

Serves 9 (4 meatballs each serving)

These Meatless Meatballs are a tasty and unique variation from the usual entree. They can be added to spaghetti dishes, cream dishes, or served plain. Nutritionally this recipe is a good buy for the money.

Soybean Stroganov

1 C. onions, sliced — *Saute* in large frypan until soft

3 C. fresh mushrooms, sliced

4 T. butter

¼ C. whole wheat flour — *Stir* in and cook 2 minutes until flour has browned

¼ C. cooking sherry — *Mix* next 6 ingredients

¾ C. water from cooked soybeans — *Stir* into above mixture and cook until thickened

2 T. boullion, beef or vegetable

2 t. Worchestershire sauce

2 t. dry mustard

dash black pepper

2 C. cooked soybeans — *Add* to sauce

1½ C. yogurt — *Stir* in immediately

before serving

Serves 6

Serve over brown rice; garnish with fresh parsley.

The Soybean Stroganov is lower in protein, iron, and the B-complex vitamins while higher in calories and cost when compared to a hamburger patty. What is the advantage of preparing this dish, you may ask?

The nutritional advantages of this recipe far outweigh the disadvantages. While it contains less protein than hamburger, the protein is of excellent quality because of the soybean content. It contains less fat calories and less saturated fat than a hamburger patty. It provides a significant contribution of carbohydrates, calcium, phosphorus, and has more vitamin A, B_1, B_2, and C than ground meat.

This meatless Stroganov recipe was considered delicious by our tasters. We recommend it as a good company dish for a vegetarian meal. Its cost could be easily lowered by decreasing the quantity of mushrooms or by using canned mushrooms instead of fresh.

Baked Bean Salad

2 C. cooked pinto beans

1 C. cheddar cheese, grated

Combine all ingredients

1 C. celery, chopped

Pour into 1½ qt. casserole dish

¼ C. onion, chopped

⅓ C. sweet pickle relish	*Bake* at 400 for 20 minutes
2 T. mayonnaise	*Serve* on top of cornchips or cornbread
1 T. soy sauce	
2 t. prepared mustard	
½ t. chili powder	*Serves* 4

The high nutritional quality and low cost of the Baked Bean Salad makes this dish even more beneficial! With the exception of protein and B_3, all nutrients either equal or surpass those in a hamburger patty. The iron content of this recipe is equal to or higher than the iron in a hamburger patty.

Normally, we depend on meat or the animal foods to supply our daily iron needs. Liver, organ meats, lean meats, and eggs are the richest sources of iron. Dark green, leafy and yellow vegetables, whole grain cereals, dried legumes, and dried fruit also contribute iron to our diets.

Many-Bean Soup

¼ C. each (all uncooked):	*Soak* 6-12 hours
red beans	*Drain*
great northern beans	
lima beans	
pinto beans	
navy beans	
lentils	
green split peas	
chick peas (garbanzos)	

7 C. water or stock	*Combine* all ingredients with beans
1 C. onions, chopped	*Cook* until beans are tender
1 C. celery, chopped	
1 C. carrots, chopped	
½ C. green pepper, chopped	
½ C. parsley, chopped	
1 clove garlic, minced	
2 bay leaves	
¼ t. each:	
marjoram	
thyme	
basil	
rosemary	
1 C. canned tomatoes, chopped	*Serves* 6

Split Pea Stew

½ C. brown rice	In crock-pot or large kettle, cover and *boil*.
6 C. liquid (broth, water)	
2 C. split peas, uncooked	*Cook* until rice is soft and peas are tender (4 hrs. in crock-pot on high; 1 hr. in kettle)
1 C. onion, chopped	
1 C. carrots, diced	*Combine* other ingredients with the above
1 C. celery, diced	
2 t. salt	*Cook* until vegetables are done
½ t. basil	

175

dash black pepper   *Serves 6*

The Many-Bean Soup and the Split Pea Stew are very high in vitamin A. Our bodies cannot synthesize this essential nutrient, so we must get it from foods we eat. The adult requirement for Vitamin A is 5000 IU a day. The Split Pea Stew provides 65% and the Many-Bean Soup provides 53% of this requirement. Both of these recipes are low in cost and calories.

The low-fat and high-carbohydrate content of both recipes make them nutritionally attractive since the majority of Americans need to make these dietary adjustments. A glass of milk added to the menu when serving the Split Pea Stew would be an excellent way to enhance the lower protein content of the stew. It would also make valuable additions to all other nutrients except iron.

The following recipes are gifts of love from the kitchens of my friends. These dishes are not only nutritious but delicious. They are a great way to introduce your family to the benefits and blessings of meatless cooking.

Eggplant Spaghetti Sauce

In large kettle, heat cup oil. Add:

1 large chopped eggplant (cut it in small pieces)

2 onions, chopped

1 green pepper, chopped

1 carrot, diced in small pieces

Saute for 15 min., stirring occasionally. Add:

2 large cans (28 oz.) tomatoes

1-15 oz. can tomato sauce (or 1 can Ragu Sauce)
1 bay leaf
2 cloves of garlic
1 t. each of basil, oregano
½ t. each of marjoram, rosemary & thyme
½ C. snipped parsley (or dry is o.k.)

Reduce heat and simmer an hour or more. Just before serving, add head finely chopped cauliflower and lb. mushrooms which have been stir-fried. Serve over whole wheat spaghetti. Serves 8 generously.

Brown Rice And Vegetables

1 C. brown rice
3 t. oil (divided)
1 C. thinly sliced carrots
3 green onions, sliced
1 med. garlic clove, crushed
1 large green pepper—cut in thin strips
1 C. thinly sliced zucchini
1 C. thinly sliced mushrooms
½ C. slivered almonds
4-5 T. soy sauce

Cook rice according to package instructions; cool. Heat 1 T. oil in skillet over high heat. Add carrots; stir about 1 minute or until carrots are almost tender. Add onions, garlic, and green pepper; stir fry 1 minute, adding more oil as needed to prevent sticking. Add zucchini, mushrooms, and almonds; stir fry about 2 minutes or until all vegetables are barely crisp-tender. Add rice and stir to break up grains and heat through. Season to taste with soy sauce. Serve at once. Serves 6.

Nutty Bulgur Pilaf

1 C. bulgur (cracked wheat)
3 T. butter
2 C. beef or chicken bouillon
2 med. carrots, shredded
½ t. salt
½ C. chopped nuts

Saute bulgur and butter in a casserole for about 5 minutes. Add all other ingredients and bring to a boil. Cover and bake at 350 for 1 hour. Serves 4.

Banana-Oatmeal-Date Cookies

2-3 bananas
1 C. chopped dates
⅓ C. oil
½ C. chopped nuts (walnuts)
½ t. salt
1 t. vanilla
1 egg (beaten)
2 C. oatmeal

Mash bananas. Add dates and oil. Mix. Add remaining ingredients. Mix. Let stand for a few minutes. Drop on greased cookie sheet and flatten. Bake at 350, 12-15 minutes. Makes 4-5 dozen.

Pecan Loaf (patties or balls)

¼ C. sunflower or sesame seeds
⅔ C. flour
1 medium onion, quartered

1 C. water
1 t. basil
1 t. salt
1 C. pecans, ground
2 C. cooked brown rice
4 C. bread crumbs, blended

Grind pecans dry in blender to make a meal. Remove from blender and mix together with rice and blended bread crumbs. Blend remaining ingredients until smooth. Combine all. Use for meatballs, patties, or as a loaf.

For loaf: pack into an oiled loaf pan and bake at 350 for 1¼ hrs.or bake in an oiled 8 x 8" pan for 60 min., uncovered. It is also good served cold, in a sandwich. Leftovers freeze well. (Makes 16 slices.)

For patties: Shape patties about ½" thick and 3" in diameter. Bake on an oiled sheet at 350 for 45 minutes.

For balls: Form balls by hand. Bake on oiled cookie sheet 40 minutes at 350.

Scrambled Tofu

1 lb. tofu, mashed
½ C. onions, chopped
2 t. dried chives
2 t. chicken style seasoning
¼ t. salt
½ t. onion powder
⅛ t. garlic powder

Saute onions in small amount of water. Add remaining ingredients, heat and serve.

For more recipes that will aid good health and help prevent disease, several good books are available.[2]

With tough love in the kitchen and God's love in your heart, you can improve your family's health by changing their eating habits. Healthy bodies that are no longer sick and tired will bring glory to God and be useful vessels for His Kingdom.

FOOTNOTES

Chapter One
1. National Livestock and Meat Board, *Food and Nutrition News,* (1978) vol. 49, p. 3.
2. Dr. Otto Schaefer, "When The Eskimo Comes to Town," *Nutrition Today*, Nov./Dec., 1971.

Chapter Two
1. Ethel Austin Martin, *Nutrition in Action,* 4th ed. (New York: Holt, Rinehart, and Winston, 1978), pp. 53-86.
2. *Ibid.*, p. 63.

Chapter Three
1. Jeffrey Bland, Ph.D., *Your Health Under Seige,*(Brattleboro, Vermont: Stephen Green Press, 1981), pp.225-226.
2. E.M.N. Hamilton and E.N. Whitney, *Nutrition Concepts and Controversies* (St. Paul: West Publishing, 1979). pp. 144-145.
3. Table 2 "Ranges of Safe Daily Intakes of the

Essential Vitamins and Minerals" from *Nutraerobics: The Complete Individualized Nutrition and Fitness Program for Life After 30,* by Jeffrey Bland, Ph.D., Reprinted by permission of Harper and Row Publishers, Inc.

Chapter Four

1. Betty Peterkin, "Bargain Hunting: Meat and Meat Alternatives," *Family Economics Review,* Fall (1978), p. 26.

2. *Family Economics Review,* Fall (1978), p. 28.

3. *Nutritive Value of American Foods in Common Units,* Handbook No. 456 (Washington, D.C.: U.S. Dept. of Agriculture, 1975).

4. E.A. Young, E.H. Bennam, and G.L. Irving, "Perspectives on Fast Foods," *Dietetic Currents,* vol. 5 (1978), p. 5.

5. E.M.N. Hamilton and E.N. Whitney, *Nutrition: Concepts and Controversies* (St. Paul: West Publishing, 1979), p. 221.

6. "It's natural! It's organic! Or is it?" *Consumer Reports,* (July, 1980), p. 10.

7. Ronald Deutsch, *Realities of Nutrition* (Palo Alto: Bull Publishing, 1976), p. 208.

Chapter Five

1. *Encyclopedia Judaica,* vol. 6 (New York: Macmillan Co., 1971), p. 1416.

2. Margaret M. Justin, Lucile Osborn Rust, and

Gladys E. Vail, *Foods* (Boston: Houghton Mifflin Co., 1956), p. 248.

3. Dr.'s Agatha and Calvin Thrash, *The Animal Connection*(Seale, Alabama: Yuchi Pines Institute, 1983), p. 10.

4. *Encyclopedia Judaica,* vol. 6, p. 40.

5. Harold P. Gastwirt, *Fraud, Corruption, and Holiness* (Port Washington, New York: Kennikat Press, 1971), p. 938.

6. *Ibid.*, p. 28,40.

7. Adam Clark, *The Holy Bible, with a commentary and critical notes,* vol. 5 (New York: Abingdon-Cokesbury Press, n.d.), p. 808.

8. *Encyclopedia Judaica,* vol. 5, p. 938.

9. William Barclay, *The Letters to the Corinthians*(Philadelphia: Westminster Press, 1954), p. 89.

10. M.E. Swendseid, "Nutritional Implications of Renal Disease," *American Dietetic Association Journal,* (1977), vol. 70, pp. 488-492.

11. A.A. Albanese and L.A. Orts, "The Proteins and Amino Acids," *Modern Nutrition in Health and Disease,* 5th ed., editors: R.S. Goodhart and M.E. Shils (Philadelphia: Lea and Febiger, 1973), pp. 28-88.

12. Barclay, *The Letters to the Corinthians,* p. 89

13. *The Universal Jewish Encyclopedia,* vol. 2 (New York: KTAV Publishing House, 1942), p. 516.

14. *Encyclopedia Judaica,* vol. 5, p. 938.
15. Used by permission of the Kansas Wheat Commission.
16. Carol Levergood, *God's Recipe.* For copies write to P.O. Box EG 936, Melbourne, Florida 32935.
17. Clark, *The Holy Bible, with a commentary and critical notes,*vol. 1, pp. 201-202.
18. *Encyclopedia Judaica,* vol. 6, p. 1418.
19. W. Corswant, *The Dictionary of Life in Bible Times* (New York: Oxford Press, 1960), p. 60.
20. *The Encyclopedia Americana,* International Edition, vol. 25 (Danbury, Connecticut: Americana Corporation, 1979), pp. 850-851.
21. Jean Mayer, *A Diet for Living* (New York: David McKay Co., 1975), p. 35.
22. Dr. George Kitzes, Dr. H.S. Schuette, and Dr. C.A. Elvehjem, "The B Vitamins in Honey," *Journal of Nutrition,* (1943), vol. 26, pp. 241-250.
23. *International Bible Dictionary* (Plainfield, New Jersey: Logos International, 1977), p. 126.

Chapter Six
1. Ann M. Crowley, *The Social and Economic Impact of Obesity*(Ann Arbor, Michigan: University Microfilms, 1977), p. 70.
2. *Ibid.,* pp. 42-70.
3. Theodore P. Labuza and A. Elizabeth Sloan,

eds., *Contemporary Nutrition Controversies* (St. Paul, Minnesota: West Publishing Co., 1979), p. 306.

4. *Ibid.*

5. Institute of Medicine, *Healthy People: The Surgeon General's Report on Health Promotion and Disease Prevention,* U.S. Dept. of Health, Education and Welfare, U.S. Govt. Printing Office, (1979), p. 30.

6. Myron Winick, ed., *Nutrition and Cancer* (New York: Wiley and Sons, 1977), p. 242.

7. Ernest L. Wynder, "Nutrition Carcinogenesis," *Food and Nutrition in Health and Disease,* (New York: New York Academy of Science Annals, 1977), vol. 300, p. 363.

8. *Ibid.*, p. 295.

9. *Nutrition Action,* Center for Science in the Public Interest, December, 1980.

10. Dr.'s Agatha and Calvin Thrash, *Nutrition For Vegetarians*(Seale, Alabama: Thrash Publications, 1982), p. 85.

11. Dr. Agatha Thrash, *The Truth About Caffeine* (Washington, D.C.: Narcotics Education, Inc.).

12. *Ibid.*

13. E. Cheraskin, W.M. Ringsdorf, J.W. Clark, *Diet and Disease*(New Canaan, Connecticut: Keats Publishing Inc., 1968), p. 58.

14. Thrash, *Nutrition For Vegetarians,* p. 52.

15. *1980 Dietary Guidelines for Americans*

(Washington, D.C.: U.S. Dept. of HEW, 1980).

Chapter Seven

1. Norris McWhirter, *1984 Guinness Book of World Records* (New York: Sterling Publishing Co.), p. 357

Chapter Eleven

1. William Barclay, *The Letters to the Galatians and Ephesians* Philadelphia: Westminster Press, 1958), pp. 164-165.
2. JoAnn Rachor, *Of These You May Freely Eat* and Dr. Agatha Thrash, *Eat For Strength.* To order write to Family Health Publications, 13062 Musgrove Highway, Sunfield, Missouri 48890.

ABOUT THE AUTHOR

Mary Ruth Swope received a Bachelor of Science degree from Winthrop College, Rock Hill, S.C., a Master of Science degree in Foods and Nutrition from the Woman's College of the University of North Carolina, Greensboro, and a doctorate from Teacher's College, Columbia University, New York City.

After seven years of high school teaching in Vocational Home Economics programs, she served as a nutritionist with the Ohio Health Department.

Dr. Swope then joined the Foods and Nutrition faculty at Purdue University and later served as Head of Foods and Nutrition at the University of Nevada.

As a college administrator, she served as Head of Home Economics at Queens College, Charlotte, N.C. For 18 years, prior to her retirement in December, 1980, Dr. Swope was Dean of the School of Home Economics, Eastern Illinois University, Charleston, Illinois.

Dr. Swope and her husband, Don, took early

retirement to begin a new ministry, "Nutrition With A Mission." Through lectures and seminars they encourage their audiences to deny themselves unneeded calories, to save the money the calories would have cost, and to give it to Great Commission programs and projects.

Dr. Swope is a popular lecturer who has been a seminar speaker at PTL in Charlotte, N.C. and Christian Retreat in Bradendon, Florida. She has also made many TV appearances including the 700 Club on the Christian Broadcasting Network.

The Swopes' current address is P.O. Box 1746, Melbourne, Florida 32901